EAT WELL, LIVE WELL

The Canadian Dietetic Association's Guide to Healthy Eating

Helen Bishop MacDonald, M.Sc., R.D.
Margaret Howard, B.Sc., R.P.Dt.

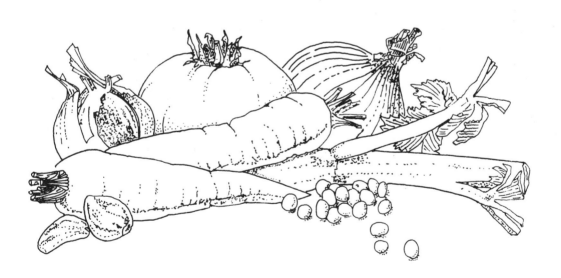

Macmillan Canada
Toronto

Canadian Cataloguing in Publication Data
MacDonald, Helen Bishop, 1939–
    Eat well, live well

ISBN 0-7715-9969-2

1. Nutrition. 2. Cookery. I. Howard, Margaret, 1930–
II. Canadian Dietetic Association. III. Title.

RM219.H68 1990   641.5′63   C90-093057-8

5 6 7 8 9 10 BP 97 96 95 94 93 92

Design and illustration: Libby Starke
Photographs: Fred Bird

Macmillan Canada
A Division of Canada Publishing Corporation
Toronto, Ontario, Canada

Printed and bound in Canada

Contents

List of photos

The Canadian Dietetic Association

The Canadian Dietetic Association is proud to bring this book to Canadians. *Eat Well, Live Well* is CDA's most comprehensive effort to date to educate Canadians about how important healthy eating is, and how easy healthy eating can be.

For the past decade, CDA has designated March as *Nutrition Month*. The goal of this campaign — the largest of its kind in Canada — is to improve eating habits of Canadians through nutrition information provided by dietitians. CDA works closely with provincial dietetic associations to ensure that more Canadians are exposed to a reliable nutrition message.

The Canadian Dietetic Association represents more than 4,500 dietitians nationwide. Founded in 1935, CDA is dedicated to the nutritional well-being of the public through its support and promotion of quality dietetic practice.

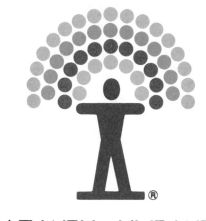

EAT WELL, LIVE WELL

T.M. The Canadian Dietetic Association

The Canadian Dietetic Association gratefully acknowledges the three official sponsors for their support of this book and the National Nutrition Campaign. The involvement of Grissol, Kellogg Canada Inc., and Kraft General Foods has been instrumental in making *Eat Well, Live Well* a reality which will help Canadians achieve a healthier lifestyle. Their participation demonstrates commitment to healthy eating and illustrates their leadership in the food industry.

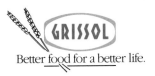

Better food for a better life.

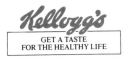

GET A TASTE
FOR THE HEALTHY LIFE

ENJOY
Nutrilicious
CHEESE

Preface

This book is like no other you have read. In it, dietitians from across Canada show you that healthy eating is fun and enjoyable, tasty and delicious. In fact, healthy eating is a true pleasure and does not require sacrifices in taste, time, or money. For easy reading and use, the book is divided into two sections: an information section and a recipe section.

The information section provides the most up-to-date facts on today's key nutrition issues. It is not intended to teach you everything you always wanted to know about nutrition: the topic is simply too vast. But it will answer some of your central questions.

For the past five years, *The Canadian Dietetic Association* has reviewed current research that examines the relationship between nutrition and diseases such as cancer, heart disease, hypertension, and obesity. We now know that diet definitely plays an important role in the prevention of these diseases, and that improving your eating habits can affect your health. The research indicates the main dietary habits that can have a positive effect on your health:

- Consume only moderate amounts of fat and fatty foods.
- Eat generous amounts of legumes, fruits, vegetables, and whole grain foods.
- Drink alcohol in moderation, if at all.
- Achieve and maintain a healthy body-fat level.
- Reduce the intake of saturated fats.
- Consume only moderate amounts of sodium.

However, the CDA has chosen to focus on four main suggestions in this book:

1. Eat a wide variety of foods.
2. Keep fat in your diet only in moderation.
3. Eat generous amounts of foods containing complex carbohydrates, and fibre.
4. Achieve and maintain a healthy weight.

These four points apply to the majority of Canadians. They are consistent with recommendations for a healthy lifestyle and for the reduction of the risk of several chronic diseases and they are achievable for most Canadians.

Nutrition is important, but it is *food* that we actually eat. The recipe section of this book provides easy and delicious ways to make healthy eating a part of your life. It is the practical application of the healthy eating message.

In 1989, The Canadian Dietetic Association sponsored a national consumer Healthy Eating recipe contest during a promotional campaign that is part of *Nutrition Month* each March across Canada. Canadians were invited to submit their favourite recipes. More than 1,200 people responded. We screened and tested the recipes, and the best ones were presented to taste panels. The results of all this testing were used to select the recipes included in this book.

Each recipe has been analyzed for nutritional content. You will find the calories, carbohydrates, protein, fat, and fibre per serving listed for each recipe. Some recipes are low in fat, others are at a medium level. A few are even high in fat. With many of the recipes, we have included menus (prepared by dietitian members of The Canadian Dietetic Association) that show you how this variety of foods can be part of healthy eating. It's all a matter of how you combine different foods in one meal and in one day. For example, if you chose one of the desserts with a higher fat content, you could balance this choice with a low-fat main course and a light salad. This combination of foods would keep your daily fat intake in check.

We certainly are not encouraging you to eat high-fat desserts every day, but a slice of chocolate cake every now and then won't hurt. We hope that this book will show you that a wide variety of foods that you normally eat and enjoy can be part of healthy eating.

So without further ado, get out your mixing bowls, try a few recipes, and *bon appetit*!

Helen Haresign, M.Sc., R.P.Dt.
Director Public Relations
The Canadian Dietetic Association

Part One | THE IMPORTANCE OF HEALTHY EATING: WHAT'S IN IT FOR YOU

"Looking good! Feeling great!" These buzz words are used to sell everything from compact cars to designer jeans. But looking good, feeling great, and performing well should begin long before you slip into those jeans or slide behind the wheel of a Ferrari. They start with good food to fuel top performance, a healthy look, that great feeling. They begin with healthy eating.

Healthy eating is simply a matter of avoiding deficiency on the one hand and avoiding excess on the other. Healthy food choices guarantee that all the vitamins, minerals, protein, fat, and carbohydrates necessary for optimum health are provided in the diet. And by "optimum health," we mean a feeling of positive well-being that is far more than simply an absence of illness or disease.

Although they are rare in North America, deficiency diseases like pellagra (niacin deficiency), beriberi (thiamin deficiency), rickets (vitamin D deficiency), or the dreaded ariboflavinosis (riboflavin deficiency) are still possible. Insufficient protein can lead to kwashiorkor, or, as it's termed in North America, adult visceral attrition. Carbohydrate insufficiency results in ketosis and, yes, you will even find fat in the list of necessary nutrients. Those overdoing the fat restriction can be left with a good case of essential fatty acid deficiency.

Minerals are also extremely important to good health, ranging from the well-known, like calcium and iron, to those the average person doesn't lose much sleep over, like molybdenum, vanadium, and tin! The beauty of it all is that the average person does not have to go out of his or her way to consume a diet balanced in all the necessary nutrients.

In North America the problem is more often too much of the wrong food rather than not enough of the right. Excess calories and fat are the most common villains, with too much salt a problem for some and excess sugar a culprit in tooth decay. Despite the increased interest in activity and exercise, many of us simply consume far more fuel than we burn, and fat accumulation is the result.

The most well-known consequence of excess body fat and too much fat in the diet is the increased risk of coronary artery disease, but there is also a suspected link between fat intake and certain forms of cancer. Obesity is associated with a greater risk of developing diabetes, high blood pressure, and gall bladder disease.

Unfortunately, the effects of poor nutrition take their toll slowly and are only noticeable in the long term. If the effects of poor eating habits were immediate, we would all be much more careful about what we put in our mouths. But because people are not always aware of the consequences of their eating habits, we must rely on education to help them understand why it's important to eat sensibly.

Many people argue that in order to eat healthily one must spend more money. Not so. In fact, the reverse is often true. Just picture some grocery carts you have seen on recent shopping trips. Frozen cakes, soft drinks, snack items, all in the cart of a shopper who is exclaiming that fresh fruit is just too expensive. What is important is that we spend our dollars on food containing lots of nutrients, rather than on those that contain mostly ''empty'' calories (that is, food rich in calories but poor in nutrients). That is not to suggest that ''fun foods'' have no place in our diets, just don't confuse money spent on empty calories with that which is spent for nutrients.

Moving from one's personal budget to that of the nation, we come to another cost of poor eating habits. The medical expenses borne by the Canadian taxpayer could be cut significantly if everyone would wake up one morning and decide to practise ''safe food habits.'' John Knowles, former president of the Rockefeller Foundation, observed that ''over 99 percent of us are born healthy and made sick as a result of personal misbehaviour and environmental conditions.'' We may frequently blame the environment for poor health, but poorly chosen food is one of the most commonplace ''personal misbehaviours'' and a very costly one, at that.

Healthy eating cannot guarantee good health. Illness and disease result from many factors. What optimum nutrition can do is give you a body that's best equipped to fend off attacks on its well-being. The importance of good nutrition is its role in risk reduction. Just as a securely fastened seat-belt offers protection against injury and death, a well-planned diet can give a definite edge in the game of life.

Four Guidelines for Healthy Eating

A complete discussion of the subject of nutrition would contain explanations of the effect of everything that finds its way into your mouth. Sodium, alcohol, caffeine, calcium, cholesterol, sugar, and food additives are but some of the substances that could be explored, but if we were that thorough, you'd need a friend to help you lift the book.

Since we can't possibly cover everything, we have chosen to focus on four main suggestions which form the basis for this book:

1. Eat a wide variety of foods.
2. Keep fat in your diet only in moderation.
3. Eat generous amounts of foods containing complex carbohydrates and fibre.
4. Achieve and maintain a healthy weight.

Healthy eating does not mean one has to become a fanatic. It doesn't have to involve strange patterns of food combinations, severe restrictions, or a general notion that if you like it, it must be bad for you. Nor does it mean that you must reject any product that hasn't come directly from your own garden. Healthy eating does not require periodic fasting or purging, nor does it insist that all bodies be pencil thin. It doesn't mean that a hamburger must never pass your lips or that birthday cakes be made from tofu. In short, healthy eating won't make a martyr out of you. On the contrary, it means keeping you around and happy for a long time.

So what is healthy eating? It is the routine choice of a variety of foods that are rich in nutrients, low in fat, and that help you maintain a healthy weight. One of the most important words in that statement is "routine." We're not discussing a perpetual vow of restraint. Instead, we recommend a pattern of eating that selects the superior and rejects the inferior. But not necessarily always. Over the next twenty years, you will consume roughly 19,000 meals. That's a lot of food. Now, you might decide on the straight and narrow for all 19,000, or you could opt for 18,000 exemplary meals and for the other 1,000, let 'er rip.

The Importance of Variety
No one food can supply all of the nutrients necessary for good health. Oh, sure, babies can thrive on just milk for a number of months, but sooner or later they need iron and vitamin C from other foods. Spinach is a great veggie, but even Popeye occasionally had something else. And even if food choices are nutritious, the same stuff day after day gets boring. One would think that natural inclination would lead people to choose a wide variety of food when it is available, but unfortunately that isn't always the case. There are those who are downright uncomfortable going beyond the range of a few familiar foods. The term "meat and potatoes man" didn't come into being by accident. It's ironic that in an age when people are adventurous enough to take up parasailing or sky-diving, they're reluctant to try eggplant. The flip side of that coin would be those who have become so concerned about nutrition that they'll only eat "health" foods. One woman who had decided to eat no animal product in any form (no meat, fish, poultry, no eggs, no milk) asked a dietitian about the adequacy of her diet. When told that she would need to take certain supplements if she adhered to this eating pattern, she replied that this could not be true since nature's foods should supply all the nutrients one needs. That's right; it should and it can. Consuming small amounts of animal products would have rounded off her diet with the necessary variety. People who focus on one or two food groups and exclude others are denying themselves the variety needed to ensure that all the bases are covered. Jack Spratt and his wife both had a problem.

In the past, fruits and vegetables were the neglected foods; nowadays, the trend has shifted, and many people, especially women, go overboard in the salad department and skimp on foods like milk and meat, so important for calcium and iron respectively.

Enter *Canada's Food Guide*. If you really want a picture of healthy eating, there it is. Simply put, the guide categorizes food into distinct groups based on their nutrient content. Then, to simplify matters even more, it makes recommendations for the number of servings to be eaten from each group each day. The recommendations cover every age and stage of life (excepting babies) for the average healthy person.

You will notice that some foods don't exactly fit into one of the food groups, especially items that are primarily fat and sugar. The guide covers these foods in a section called "Moderation," which basically means it's not necessary to reject them entirely, just be careful.

Even by following the guide to the letter, however, it's possible to lack sufficient variety. Take, for example, a diet consisting of the following: milk, chicken, carrots, and pasta. Each is a food from one of

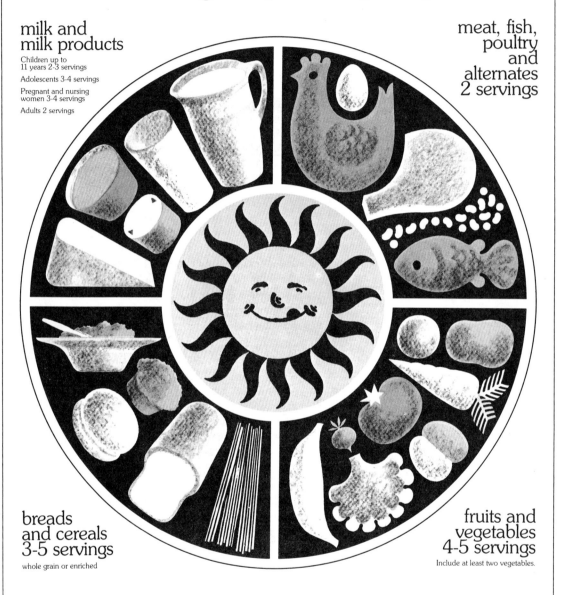

Canada's Food Guide

Eat a variety of foods from each group every day

milk and milk products

Children up to 11 years 2-3 servings

Adolescents 3-4 servings

Pregnant and nursing women 3-4 servings

Adults 2 servings

meat, fish, poultry and alternates 2 servings

breads and cereals 3-5 servings

whole grain or enriched

fruits and vegetables 4-5 servings

Include at least two vegetables.

Health and Welfare Canada   Santé et Bien-être social Canada

Canadä

the food groups, but eating nothing but those four would obviously not be the path to healthy eating. That's an exaggeration to make a point—it's unlikely that anyone would be so limited in their food choices—but for some it's not much of an exaggeration.

Variety and moderation go together; they make up a handy little nutrition motto: *a variety of foods taken in moderation makes for healthy eating.*

Fat Intake in Moderation

Probably no nutrient has received as much attention in the history of nutrition as fat. Actually, that's not quite true. Remember when starch was a four-letter word? Despite dietitians' efforts to convince them otherwise, many people believed that the root cause of obesity was found in potatoes, bread, and pasta. How times have changed.

The main difference between carbohydrate-chaos and fat-furore is that dietitians did not support the rejection of carbohydrates, but now they are actively trying to persuade folks to reduce their intake of fat. The typical Canadian gets roughly 40 percent of the calories in his or her diet from fat. Dietitians and health agencies recommend that people aim for no more than 30 percent of the calories in their diet from fat. Nutrition research has indicated that a number of medical problems are related to excessive fat intake, among them heart disease, obesity, and certain forms of cancer. More specifically, diets rich in saturated fats have been associated with elevated blood cholesterol levels. Therefore, among the most important, if not the most important dietary prescriptions for Canadians is to lower their consumption of fat.

What needs to be pointed out is that *every* fat or oil—whether it comes from a pig or a parsnip—contains nine calories per gram. Some people feel quite proud of having "only" a Caesar salad for lunch. When cautioned about the oil in it, they reply that it's all right, since it is a vegetable oil! Too much fat is too much fat, regardless of the type.

Fat is a powerhouse of energy compared to protein and carbohydrate, which each carry only four calories per gram. Gram for gram, therefore, fat contributes more than twice as much energy (calories) as carbohydrate or protein. One needn't be a rocket scientist to figure out what this does to our overall girth. In addition, some scientists have shown that calories from fat become part of our body fat more easily than calories from carbohydrate or protein. Since fat is a large part of many popular food items, the healthy eater must be aware of the sources of fat and methods of reducing fat intake. This book will help you do just that.

Making the challenge even more interesting is the fact that, although all fats are equally high in calories, they are not all created equal. Dietary fats consist of three basic types: saturated, polyunsaturated, and monounsaturated.

Saturated fats are those that are solid at room temperature, plus (by some quirk of nature) coconut oil and palm kernel oil. Most of them come from animal sources such as milk fat (including cheese, butter, and cream), egg yolks, and the fat in meat, but vegetable oils can be hydrogenated (we'll clear up "hydrogenated" in a minute) to become saturated.

Diets rich in saturated fats have been associated with elevated blood cholesterol levels. These, in turn, have been shown to increase the risk of coronary artery disease.

Polyunsaturates are liquid at room temperature. Sources of polyunsaturated fats include safflower oil, sunflower oil, corn oil, and soybean oil.

Monounsaturates are also liquid at room temperature and are found in nuts, olive oil, and canola oil.

To help you get a handle on the differences among the saturates, polys, and monos, picture a baseball diamond. If the four bases each hold hydrogen, we could say that the bases are loaded or *saturated* with hydrogen. If you remove hydrogen from one base, you have one empty base. "Mono" means one, hence the term "monounsaturate." Remove hydrogens from two or more bases and you have a "polyunsaturate."

Now suppose you wanted to make a polyunsaturated vegetable oil (a liquid) resemble a solid saturated fat like butter or lard. What would you do? Well, you would add hydrogen, which would give you another type of fat that's almost as saturated as the real McCoy: "hydrogenated" vegetable oil, another important name to remember. It refers to vegetable oils that have had hydrogens added so that they are saturated like butter. Margarine is an example. One difference with these oils is that unlike butter and lard they contain no cholesterol. No plant product contains cholesterol: nuts don't have it, avocados don't have it. Even coconut oil doesn't contain cholesterol, although it is a saturated fat. Only animal products contain cholesterol.

And Speaking of Cholesterol . . .

Cholesterol is a fatty substance in our blood that is needed to form hormones, cell membranes, and other substances. This blood cholesterol is produced in the liver. Some cholesterol is good, but problems arise when the blood levels get too high. Elevated blood cholesterol is a major risk factor associated with the development of heart disease. By choosing a diet that is reduced in fat, emphasizes polyunsaturates and monounsaturates, and includes generous amounts of complex carbohydrates, you are making a positive step in controlling blood cholesterol levels.

Cholesterol is also found in some of the foods we eat, such as egg yolks, liver and other organ meats, shrimp and some other seafood, and in the animal fats mentioned earlier. We call this "dietary cholesterol." However, the amount of cholesterol you eat is not as significant a factor as the total amount of fat, as well as saturated fat, in your diet.

The important thing is to limit the intake of all fat but not to the point of exclusion. Fat is our only source of essential fatty acids and acts as a carrier for the fat-soluble vitamins A, D, E, and K.

A fat-reduced diet can be tasty and not that difficult to follow. Simply be aware of the various sources of fat.

A word of caution here. While most adults' diets could do with a little fat reduction, children under the age of two should not be unduly restricted. Some infants have even been hospitalized because their growth was stunted by their well-intentioned but misdirected parents' strict nutrition practices. The children's milk had to be skim, no snacking was allowed, nor was red meat permitted. This overreaction to bits of nutritional truths endangered the children's health.

On the other hand, there is a great deal of evidence that coronary artery disease begins early in life. So children, and the adults they will be one day, do benefit from a diet that keeps fat in moderation. If nothing else, it will help them form good dietary habits that will stand them in good stead later in life.

Establishing a good diet for children isn't all that difficult. Healthy eating for kids doesn't mean no ice cream, no pizza, no hamburgers. It means making sure they get a variety of the "basics" (milk, meat, grains, fruit, and vegetables) and go easy on the "extras" (fats, cakes and cookies, candies, and greasy snacks).

At this point we're still talking about homemade burgers and pizzas, but there's hope that even fast-food restaurants will respond to consumer demands for fat reduction. (Did you ever think you'd get a salad at a hamburger joint?) Healthy eating doesn't mean a family must never darken the doorway of a fast-food restaurant. But if these fast foods are eaten often, then the rule of thumb should be to choose the lower-fat items: a smaller hamburger, milk instead of a shake, and a salad, without blobs of salad dressing, instead of fries.

Fat Attack

How can you tell if you are eating the right amount of fat? We recommend that no more than 30 percent of the calories in your diet be derived from fat. But how in heaven's name can you calculate and apply these figures to your daily bread, or bacon, as the case may be?

Easy. Get out a pencil and paper and follow along. Suppose, for the sake of this discussion, that your daily intake is 2,000 calories. Thirty percent of that would give you $2000 \times 0.30 = 600$. So you want no more than 600 calories from fat. Remembering that each gram of fat yields 9 calories, we divide 600 by 9 and get 66 grams of fat (okay, so it's 66.666, but we're trying to keep this simple).

Here we are with 66 grams of fat at our disposal. So far, so good, but now we need a benchmark to get a handle on "grams of fat." Let's take the little squares of butter served in restaurants. These pats contain roughly 4 grams of fat. If you were going to eat all of the fat in your diet as butter, you could have 16 ½ pats per day. But then nothing else that passed your lips could contain any fat. Some butter fanciers might opt for that arrangement; but most others might decide to vary the sources of fat in their diet. Let's look at those other sources.

The Dairy Case

Milk products are out of favour with some people these days because they contain saturated fats. It's true, they do, but they are also extremely rich in many important nutrients: calcium, protein, and riboflavin to name but a few. Consider 2 percent, 1 percent, skim, and buttermilk. All these choices contribute the same important nutrients, but the fat in them has been reduced.

The beauty of milk products is that their fat content is listed on the label. Unfortunately, some of us need help to interpret the information.

Let's take cheddar cheese as an example. The label says 31 percent M.F. (for milk fat) or maybe B.F. (for butter fat). That tells us that if we had 100 grams of cheese (a little over 3 ounces), 31 grams would be fat. Some skim-milk mozzarellas are available at 15 percent M.F. and there are even a few hard cheeses at 7 percent, or only 7 grams of fat out of 100. Yoghurts come with the same handy information, all the way from 0.05 percent M.F. up to "rich and creamy" 8 percent M.F. Sour cream comes in varying amounts of fat, and one can even get "light" butter and margarine, in which some of the fat has been replaced by buttermilk or water. Making smart choices can add up to some real fat savings.

- Choose 2 percent, 1 percent, skim or buttermilk.
- Compare labels for M.F. (milk fat) or B.F. (butter fat) to determine fat content.
- Use milk instead of cream or "whitener" in your coffee.

The Bakery

More difficult to compute than the fat in milk is that found in commercially made baked goods. Plain breads have only a trace of fat, and rolls and bagels check in at 2 grams, but a croissant is laden with 12 grams.

Cereals are traditionally another good choice with only a trace of fat. The big exception is granola, which can add up to 15 grams of fat per bowl.

Choose your crackers wisely. Select crackers that are low in fat like melba toast and rusks. Go easy on the fancy snack crackers that are prepared with more fat.

- Read labels and choose products with lower fat, for example, bran flakes instead of granola, melba toast instead of crackers.
- Choose baked goods with lower fat content, for example, plain breads, rolls, and bagels instead of croissants, donuts, or danish.

The Produce Section

Fruits and vegetables are excellent low-fat choices. The only exception is the avocado, which boasts 25 grams of fat accompanying its other nutrients.

- Choose and serve vegetables without rich sauces.

The Meat Counter

It's not easy to calculate the amount of fat in meat, hence the admonition to buy meat as lean as possible, to trim off all visible fat before cooking, and to avoid cooking it in added fat. Meat, like milk products, is one source of fat, but it is also a nutrient-dense food loaded with B vitamins, iron, and zinc.

Processed meats are often found in Canadian refrigerators; more and more of these products are appearing with a reduced fat content. Again the percentages are noted on the label (of the fat-reduced products), giving us ham at less than 5 percent fat, as an example. One ounce of regular ham could provide 5 grams of fat and 70 calories; the fat-reduced variety has only 1.5 grams of fat and 27 calories.

- Choose lean cuts.
- Trim off visible fat before cooking.
- Instead of gravy, flavour meat with natural juices.
- Bake, broil, microwave, or roast meat on a rack instead of frying.
- Serve small portions.

Oils and Dressings
A tablespoon (15 mL) of any oil contains 14 grams of fat. Other sources of fat are mayonnaise, mayonnaise "types," and salad dressings. Real mayonnaise has 11 grams of fat per tablespoon; the imitations come in around 6. Food manufacturers have responded to consumer demand for low-fat products, and we now have "salad-type dressings" with as little as 2 grams of fat per tablespoon. Oil-free salad dressings are available with 0.2 grams of fat per tablespoon. Not all "light" dressings are equally reduced in fat, so read the label.

The "Visible" Fats
Butter and margarine contain the same amount of fat and the same number of calories. Both provide 11 grams of fat and 100 calories per tablespoon.

- Use a non-stick pan to decrease fat needed for frying.
- Use paper liners in muffin tins, rather than greasing the tins.
- Use less butter or margarine; try the "light" variety.
- Use less mayonnaise and dressings; try the "light" kind.
- Avoid deep frying.

More Suggestions for Reducing Fat
- Choose low-fat snacks like unbuttered popcorn or pretzels instead of greasy snacks.
- Make cream sauces with milk instead of cream.
- Save rich desserts for very special occasions, or share with a friend.
- Use herbs and spices to add flavour to food, rather than rich sauces and gravies.

Complex Carbohydrates and Fibre:
What It Is and Where to Find It
If people are going to decrease the amount of fat in their diets, then obviously they should and will have to replace it with something. What then should that something be? Gummy bears? Not exactly.

What we all should consume in greater quantities are complex carbohydrates, or complex carbs, as the "in" set call them. These are found in many different foods: fruits and vegetables, grains, cereals, beans, breads, rice, pasta. The variety is almost endless. In the recipe section you will find new and interesting ways of serving complex carbohydrates that are not only good for you, but delicious, too.

Hand in glove with most complex carbohydrates comes another important ingredient in your diet, and that's fibre. But let's begin at the beginning.

The terms "light" and "lite" are being used on many product labels and ads. You might assume that the term means calorie reduced. However, that is not always the case.

"Light" can be used to describe caloric content, but can also be used to describe other characteristics such as colour, texture, body, taste, sugar, alcohol, fat, etc.

Just What Is a Carbohydrate?

Carbohydrate means carbon, hydrogen, and oxygen. A carbohydrate that has one carbon unit for each group of two hydrogens and one oxygen is said to be a monosaccharide. Glucose and fructose are both examples of monosaccharides, or simple sugars. Now, if you take two monosaccharides and bond them together, things get a little less simple and you get a disaccharide. Thus, the union of glucose and fructose gives you sugar (sucrose). If you really get carried away with the process and combine many monosaccharides, you end up with a polysaccharide, otherwise referred to as a ''starch.''

Now there's a twist in the plot. Depending on how the monosaccharides are joined together, they may or may not be able to be broken down by the body's enzymes. Cellulose, a component of the walls of plant cells, is an example of an indigestible polysaccharide. Wheat bran cereals are a popular source of cellulose. A close cousin is hemicellulose. Both these fibres or indigestible polysaccharides are non-water-soluble, something that has a great bearing on their function in the body (we'll discuss this shortly). Then we have water-soluble fibres, like the gums found in oat bran and legumes, and the pectin in fruits and vegetables.

Lignin is, for the purposes of our discussion, the final type of fibre, and it isn't even a carbohydrate. Lignins are actually polymers of aromatic alcohols. Relax, we won't get into that, but you should know that the older a plant is, the more lignin it contains. Bite into an old parsnip for an illustration of this type of fibre.

You get the picture. The term ''fibre'' refers to five types of substances in plants. The one thing they all have in common is that you can't digest them. What's in them for you? Well, let's look more closely, first at the non-water-soluble fibres.

Insoluble Fibres

Non-water-soluble fibres help keep you ''regular.'' They do this by swelling up with water and producing more and softer stools. Of course, they can't swell up with water if there isn't enough water there to begin with, hence the importance of increased fluid consumption along with increased fibre intake. Not only will these fibres increase stool bulk, they also reduce the amount of time that waste matter spends hanging around the colon. Some scientists have speculated that it's possible that this rapid transit might play a part in reducing one's chances of getting cancer of the colon. Note ''possible''—not proven. Other nasty diseases that have been linked to a low intake of the non-water-soluble fibres include diverticular disease and hemorrhoids. In fact, it was the very low incidence of these diseases in cultures with a high fibre intake that first interested Dr. Denis Burkitt, a pioneer in the field of fibre research.

We still don't know for sure that it's the fibres in the diet that offer the protection. It may be that people who consume generous amounts of fibre get a healthy dose of important nutrients along with it, or that when there's a lot of fibre in the diet there's usually less fat. But whichever way you look at it, healthy eating has to include a variety of fibre-rich foods.

Soluble Fibre

There is some evidence that the water-soluble fibres, pectin and gums, may help lower blood cholesterol levels and keep blood sugar levels under control. Some fruits and vegetables are excellent sources of pectin, and the best-known source of gum is oat bran. This cereal has taken North America by storm, and the claims actually have some basis in science. The danger is that some people figure they can eat all the fat they want if they just start the day off with oat bran. This is definitely not true. But it is true that on a fat-restricted diet, a significant level of soluble fibre may help lower cholesterol levels.

Another important source of fibre is the lowly bean, which hasn't received nearly the attention that oat bran has, but is nonetheless an excellent food. We're one of the few cultures in the world that doesn't eat beans as a staple in our diet, which is most unfortunate. Beans that are a source of soluble fibre include kidney beans, lima beans, pinto beans, and white beans — all the legume kinds of beans. They don't include the green and yellow beans. These are good foods, but not great sources of soluble fibre.

Can You Have Too Much of a Good Thing?

All this is not to suggest that one must become a fibre fanatic. The typical Canadian diet contains roughly half the fibre it should, so most of us have a long way to go before we're eating too much fibre. Canadians currently eat about 15 grams of fibre a day. It has been recommended that Canadians should aim to double this amount to approximately 30 grams daily. Still, excessive consumption of anything, including fibre, is not a good idea. Bouts of diarrhea and gas will likely accompany a sudden jump onto the bran wagon. You can avoid this undesirable effect by increasing your intake gradually to the recommended level. In addition, too much fibre — or the substances that accompany it, like oxalic acid and phytic acid — may impede absorption of minerals. In other words, if you consume too much fibre, you might come up short in the calcium, iron and zinc department. You can avoid these undesirable effects by increasing your intake gradually.

A really big word of caution goes to those who would put an end to irregularity by the use of chemical-type laxatives. Too often people get hooked on them, and their bowels forget their original job description. Nature provided us with a pretty good system. Regular maintenance, however, is the responsibility of the body owner. Insoluble fibre is an important part of that maintenance.

Assuming, then, that you're convinced of the importance of fibre, how can you best adjust your diet to get a generous amount?

Finding the Fibre

One of the earliest reference to fibre was in the sixth century B.C. Pythagoras took his mind off right-angled triangles long enough to proclaim that people should avoid beans. A few centuries later, Hippocrates compounded the error by stating that people should eat white bread rather than whole grain since it produces less feces. Times have changed.

The first step in increasing your fibre intake is knowing where to find it. And perhaps the best way to illustrate where fibre is, is to tell you where it isn't. You won't find it in meat or milk products. That's it. All other basic food commodities, in varying degrees, will contribute one or more of the various fibres to your diet. The trick is to make the best choice and to consume a variety of foods containing different types of fibre.

Let's take bread as an example. As maligned as white bread is, it's not completely worthless. It is a source of complex carbohydrates and does have added B vitamins and iron. What it lacks, along with trace minerals, is fibre. Any whole grain bread — whole wheat, whole rye or any of the multi-grain combinations — is a far superior choice. So the very first step in your fibre program should be to go for the whole grain — that is, a grain or cereal from which the outer bran layer hasn't been removed.

This approach applies equally to cereals. Reading the package label tells you cereals are a source of B vitamins and iron, as well as complex carbs. If you're interested in fibre, look for whole grain ingredients and read the nutrition label for the fibre content. The real powerhouses of fibre in the cereal world are, of course, those that contain a large proportion of bran (the outer coat of the cereal grain seed). But remember that all brans are not created equal: wheat bran is primarily a source of the non-water-soluble fibres, oat bran of water-soluble fibres. You may choose to make bran muffins out of raw bran, but it is not too appetizing on its own, so you'd hardly want to eat it all by itself as a cereal. Some people choose to sprinkle a couple of tablespoons of it over other, more palatable cereals.

Nowadays there are lots of interesting cereals and grains available. Bulgur, millet, buckwheat, groats, and couscous are a few you might want to try. The recipe section of the book presents some tasty recipes using these grains.

A potential source of fibre in the typical Canadian diet is the starch source in the meal. Every culture has it: whether it is pasta, rice, potatoes, or poi, there is usually starch in some form or other. Unfortunately, we usually go out of our way to de-fibre it. The potato is actually a pretty good source of fibre, especially if you leave the skin on, and it's a terrific source of nutrients, potassium and vitamin C, for instance. As we've become more cosmopolitan, however, the potato is often pushed off the plate in favour of rice or pasta. This is okay, except that the rice and pasta are usually of the denuded, white variety. Instant rice, polished rice, even long-grain converted rice are essentially in the same category as white bread. Yes, they are a source of nutrients and complex carbohydrates but not the terrific source of fibre that brown rice is. There is even whole-grain rice available now that cooks in only 25 minutes, as opposed to the 45 minutes brown rice normally takes. Remember, too, that the bran of brown rice is an excellent source of soluble fibre.

While white rice and white pasta are fine sources of complex carbohydrates, they aren't great at providing fibre. So enjoy your dish of spaghetti or fettucine primavera, but if it's fibre you're after, look for whole wheat pasta. If you're having white pasta, serve it with a fibre source like chopped broccoli. The recipe for Pasta with Broccoli Herb Sauce (page 172) illustrates this combo.

Beans, the Unsung Heroes

One surefire way to increase your fibre intake is with dried peas and beans, members of the legume family. Usually when Canadians think "beans," they think of canned baked beans. These are okay — if you don't eat the piece of fat — but there's a whole world of beans out there waiting to be sampled. Black beans, black-eyed peas, garbanzos or chick peas, kidney beans, lentils, lima beans, pinto beans, white and navy beans, and split peas should get you started.

Beans are an excellent source of protein, but it's incomplete protein, meaning that they don't contain the complete mixture of amino acids that our bodies need. Amino acids are the building blocks of protein, and certain ones need to be included in our diet in the right proportions. That incompleteness can be remedied easily by serving other complementary incomplete proteins like rice (do you suppose the early Mexicans knew a dietitian?), or whole wheat bread, or with a bit of complete protein, like lean meat. The recipe section has some great combination dishes.

Beans are a rich source of B vitamins and also supply calcium, magnesium, phosphorus, and potassium. And, of course, the fibre. Also, relatively speaking, they're cheap.

Beans don't have to be dull, either. Aside from baking them, they can be pureed for a dip, mashed, molded, or mixed and made into casseroles, soups, or salads.

One final word: "canned" isn't synonymous with "bad for you." Many varieties of canned beans are available without any added fat, particularly pinto beans and chick peas. Refried beans usually contain fat, but you can mash a can of pinto beans and fry them up in a little olive oil or canola oil, toss in a few jalapenos — ole! The point is, if you get home from work tired and hungry, opening up a can of beans isn't a bad thing. Add some sliced tomatoes or salad, some whole wheat bread, and a glass of low fat milk — there's healthy eating.

Even more exotic than some of the beans mentioned is a garbanzo bean product quickly gaining in popularity — falafel. This Middle Eastern "fast food" is made from mashed garbanzos, seasoned and cooked as patties or balls. They are great stuffed into a pita pocket with some tomatoes, sprouts, lettuce, and a little yoghurt. Garbanzos also make an appearance in another dish from the Middle East — hummus. This dish also includes tahini, or sesame seed paste, which is another source of fibre. The recipe section will help you cook up both these dishes.

Speaking of sesame seeds brings us to the nuts and seeds sources of fibre. Along with fibre, nuts and seeds contribute many important nutrients, such as B vitamins and minerals. They also contribute fat, however, so go easy. There's no such thing as a low-cal peanut butter.

Fibre in Fruits and Vegetables

Now that you're full of beans, let's look at another fibre source: fruits and vegetables.

While all fruits are good sources of fibre, some are better than others. Topping the list are dates, figs, and prunes. Canadians, sadly, often think of prunes as something for the elderly, dates as only found in squares, and figs in cookies. Yet these fruits make great snacks for people who

FIBRE COMPARISON: HOW DOES YOUR DAY STACK UP?

Low Fibre Day

BREAKFAST
4 oz. (125 mL) grapefruit juice
2 slices white toast
2 pats butter
2 tsp. (10 mL) jam
8 oz. (250 mL) milk

LUNCH
2 slices white bread
2 oz. (60 g) tuna
mayonnaise
lettuce
8 oz. (250 mL) milk
chocolate pudding

DINNER
roast chicken
mashed potatoes
creamed corn
lettuce salad
8 oz. (250 mL) milk
brownies

High Fibre Day

BREAKFAST
1/2 grapefruit
1 slice whole wheat toast
1 tbsp. (15 mL) peanut butter
oatmeal or bran cereal
8 oz. (250 mL) milk

LUNCH
2 slices rye bread
2 oz. (60 g) tuna
mayonnaise
tomato slices
shredded cabbage
8 oz. (250 mL) milk
fruit salad

DINNER
chili with kidney beans
shredded carrot/zucchini
  salad
cornbread
8 oz. (250 mL) milk
sunflower seed cookies

want more fibre and no fat. They aren't a tooth's best friend, however; so brush afterwards.

Fresh fruits taste better than canned, but are not always available. The problem with canned fruits is not that the fibre is destroyed—it isn't—but many products have a sugary syrup that increases calories. Buy those packed in their own juice. Frozen fruits without added sugar are becoming more plentiful and are an excellent choice in winter.

Some vegetables are surprisingly low in fibre—lettuce, celery, and onions are examples. For the most part, however, vegetables make an important fibre contribution and are extremely low in fat.

To sum up then, many health organizations have stressed the importance of eating more complex carbohydrates and emphasizing a variety of fibre-rich choices, including whole-grain breads and cereals, fruits and vegetables, beans and nuts.

If you plan to increase your fibre consumption, it is important to do it gradually and increase your fluid intake at the same time. Otherwise you are likely to encounter some unpleasant side effects, like gas or diarrhea.

Practical Suggestions for Increasing Fibre in Your Diet

Bread: choose whole wheat, rye, pumpernickel, multi-grain.

Cereals: select those with whole grain ingredients or bran—wheat, oat, corn, and rice.

Crackers: pick whole wheat or rye, rice crackers made from brown rice.

Rolls and muffins: choose whole wheat, bran, or oat bran, but beware —some commercial products are often high in fat.

Pasta: try whole grain, or at least add a fibrous vegetable if you are serving white pasta.

Rice: substitute brown for white; try brown rice in casseroles that call for pasta.

Fruits and vegetables: when possible, eat fruits and vegetables with the skin or peel left on—whole products have more fibre than juice does.

Legumes: increase your consumption of kidney beans, split peas, lentils, chick peas, and so forth.

Soups and casseroles: add vegetables and legumes to soups and casseroles; use oatmeal and other cereals, wheat germ, nuts, seeds.

Baking: when white flour is called for, substitute whole wheat for part or all of the flour.

A Healthy Weight: There Is a Way Out of the Diet Maze

Weight is a national obsession. We are bombarded with images of thinness. Flipping through magazines at the newspaper stand, what do you see? Promises of a great body in 10 days, quicky diets, and skinny models. A mammoth industry now thrives on our North American obsession with trim waistlines. Each year millions are spent on diet clinics and books, reducing aids, exercise classes, and diet foods. Nevertheless, many Canadians are still overweight and suffer from weight-related conditions. Others, especially women, believe they are overweight when they aren't. Our obsession has led to a growing number of health problems associated with weight loss, radical dieting, and being underweight.

Healthy Weight: What's It All About?

Your body weight does have an effect on your health. Both overweight and underweight people are at higher risk for health problems. Carrying an excessive amount of body fat puts an extra strain on the heart, the circulatory system, and many of the body's organs, which can lead to chronic illnesses. The important thing is to know what is a healthy weight for you, and if you're above or below the acceptable range, to find a suitable, healthy diet to help you reach that weight.

Body Mass Index

The goal now is to redirect our thinking away from an obsession with weight to a concern with a healthy body size and the right proportion of body fat. Body fat is the problem, not a particular weight. Canadians have been so conditioned by the term "weight" and what it tells them about the acceptability of their bodies that many have become slaves to the bathroom scale and the magic number revealed there. But the term "weight" can be very misleading. A weight scale reports the pull of gravity on a mass. Period. That mass might be bone, muscle, water, fat, or, in the case of the body, a combination of all four.

With that in mind, Canadians are urged to begin thinking in terms of a different measure—the Body Mass Index or BMI.

$$\text{BMI} = \frac{\text{Weight (in kilograms)}}{\text{Height (in metres)}^2}$$

Small, tall, sturdy, delicate—great bodies come in all sizes. Now with the BMI, you can see if your present size falls into the healthy weight zone. After all, it's our health that we want for years to come.

To find your BMI, take your weight in kilograms (pounds divided by 2.2) and divide it by your height in metres (inches × 0.025), squared. Don't panic; you don't have to be Einstein to do this—although a calculator does help. Suppose your height is 5'4" or 64 inches. Multiply that by 0.025 to give you 1.6 metres. To square that, simply multiply it by itself to get 2.56. So then, supposing your weight is 120 pounds or 54.5 kilograms, your BMI is 54.5 divided by 2.56, which is 21.3. Terrific—but now what do you do with that number?

Easy. Check the chart on the next page. If your BMI is lower than 20 or higher than 25, you are not at a healthy weight. Below 20 means you could use a little more mass on your bones, and over 25 tells you that some fat loss is probably in order. Note the term "fat loss." It will be a major breakthrough in attitude when people replace the term "weight loss" with "fat loss." Weight isn't the point.

BMI is designed for the average, healthy adult. It is not intended to calculate the healthy weights of children, adolescents, pregnant women, seniors, or athletes. It's not perfect, but it does serve as a guide for people interested in maintaining a healthy weight.

The promotion of healthy weights for all Canadians is an important issue. The healthy weight concept requires a positive attitude change for increased tolerance of a variety of body shapes and sizes.

HOW TO FIND YOUR BMI – IT'S EASY

1. Mark an X at your height on line A.
2. Mark an X at your weight on line B.
3. Take a ruler and join the two X's.
4. To find your BMI, extend the line to line C.

FOR EXAMPLE:

- If Michael is 1.80 m (5'11") and weighs 85 kg (188 lbs), his BMI is about 26.
- If Irene is 1.60 m (5'4") and weighs 60 kg (132 lbs), her BMI is about 23.

Under 20 A BMI under 20 may be associated with health problems for some individuals. It may be a good idea to consult a dietitian and physican for advice.

20-25 This zone is associated with the lowest risk of illness for most people. This is the range you want to stay in.

25-27 A BMI over 25 may be associated with health problems for some people. Caution is suggested if your BMI is in this zone.

Over 27 A BMI over 27 is associated with increased risk of health problems such as heart disease, high blood pressure and diabetes. It may be a good idea to consult a dietitian and physician for advice.

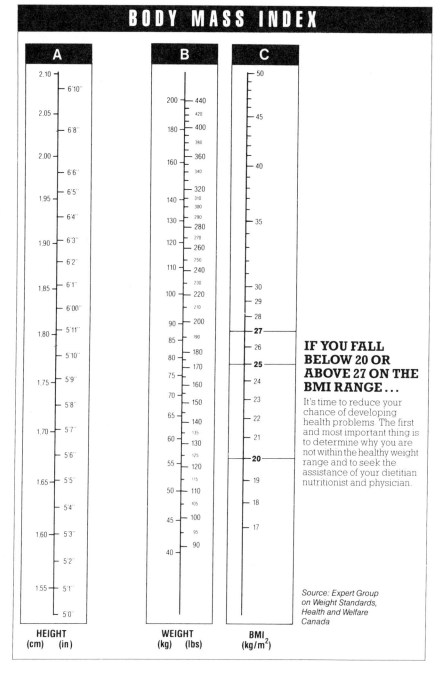

IF YOU FALL BELOW 20 OR ABOVE 27 ON THE BMI RANGE...

It's time to reduce your chance of developing health problems. The first and most important thing is to determine why you are not within the healthy weight range and to seek the assistance of your dietitian nutritionist and physician.

Source: Expert Group on Weight Standards, Health and Welfare Canada

The Relationship Between Your Waist and Hips

But let's not stop there. It's been shown that not only is the total body fat content a significant factor in health, but the pattern of fat distribution is important as well. Too much fat around the waist, most typical of men, is associated with high blood pressure and cardiovascular illness. Women, on the other hand, tend to deposit fat a bit lower down and in the thigh area.

To help determine the pattern of fat deposition, a form of assessment called the Waist to Hip Ratio has been developed. Relax. This one's a cinch. Simply divide your waist measurement by your hip measurement. If the answer is greater than 1.0 and you're male, then you want to lose some fat; for women the number is anything more than 0.8.

The important thing to remember is that you're aiming for a healthy weight, not to be the skinniest person on your block. Healthy eating and exercising will make you trimmer and keep you fit, but there's no changing what you were born with. You inherited your body build; keep it in shape, so you can always feel your best.

Be A Wise Loser

If you've ever had a spell of diarrhea and weighed yourself afterwards, you may have noticed a loss of up to five pounds. Five pounds of what? Water. And perhaps some muscle and some fat. Within a week you were most likely back to your pre-illness weight.

Water loss, however, can mean big business. One of the major problems with some of the commercial get-slim-quick schemes is that in their desire to meet the rapid weight loss demanded by clients, they put people on a severely restricted caloric intake, which naturally results in impressive "weight" loss. But again the question is raised: what kind of weight? Some fat, certainly, but also significant amounts of muscle and water. After the diet, the body will automatically replace the lost fluids, but lost muscle won't be regained unless the person goes on a muscle-building program. Worst of all, because of the low energy level of some of these diets, the body reduces its basal metabolic rate (the basic amount of energy needed to keep you ticking), and when food consumption increases even to 1,000 calories, fat is quickly redeposited. Moreover, during this quick weight loss period, the dieter hasn't developed any new good habits to ensure he or she doesn't regain the lost body fat.

The moral of this story is that if you need to lose some fat to be in a healthy range, pick a safe and sensible program. Take a careful look at the diet you're being offered, whether in a magazine or at a weight-control clinic. Ask the following questions:

1. Does the diet include foods you normally eat and enjoy?
2. Does it include a variety of foods from all four food groups?
3. Does it include enough food choices to meet the serving recommendations of Canada's Food Guide?
4. Does the diet rely on food, rather than pills or meal replacements, to provide essential nutrients?
5. Does the diet recommend an increase in physical activity?
6. Does it provide a gradual weight loss of about 1 kilogram (2 pounds) per week?

7. Are you allowed snacks?
8. Does the diet recommend a variety of foods and not promote any one food?
9. Do you think you could follow the diet for a long period of time?
10. Does the diet suggest that you consult a doctor?

The answers to all ten questions should be yes. Here's a question-by-question analysis of the reasons:

1. If the diet includes a variety of foods you normally eat and enjoy, you are more likely to stick with it and enjoy it for a period of time.
2. Including foods from all four food groups—milk and milk products; meat, fish, poultry and alternates; fruits and vegetables; breads and cereals—ensures variety and a good balance of nutrients.
3. If the foods you select follow the recommendations of Canada's Food Guide, then your body is probably getting all the essential nutrients. Thin body or fat body, both require the same nutrients, just a different number of calories.
4. There are more than 50 nutrients that your body requires to function efficiently. Read the label on the vitamin bottle or meal replacement can; how many nutrients are missing? A pill or powder has no special power to reduce weight. It is only a sign that something is lacking in the diet that it accompanies.
5. The best weight-loss program recommends decreasing the number of calories you eat and increasing the calories you burn up in activity. Find activities you enjoy and participate in them for a minimum of 20 minutes, at least 3 times per week.
6. If a diet allows rapid weight loss (more than 2 pounds per week), it is probably too low in calories for you and is unlikely to provide all the essential nutrients. This type of diet can result in loss of water and muscle tissue instead of just fat. A diet too low in calories is also difficult to follow for very long, because you feel tired, hungry, and deprived. It is usually very difficult to stick to in everyday social situations. Your weight was gained gradually, not 10 pounds in a week, and it needs to come off the same way.
7. Snacking is a way of life for most people. Including snacks in a diet helps relieve hunger and is useful in social situations.
8. There is no one food or combination of foods that has any "miraculous power" to take away fat, not even grapefruit.
9. If a diet sounds appealing enough to follow for a long period of time, you are more likely to stick to it and be successful in your weight-loss program.
10. It is always a good idea to talk to your doctor before going on a weight-loss program. He or she can advise you whether weight reduction could aggravate or precipitate any medical condition.

(*Reprinted with permission from The Ontario Dietetic Association, 1985.*)

Choose good-tasting foods and eat well, exercise regularly but not excessively and make the best of what you've got. Feel good about yourself. Beauty, the right attitude, and health go hand in hand.

Life-Styles and Food-Styles of Today

Many people today live mainly in the "fast lane" with little time for the traditional sit-down meal. But this new mode of living doesn't necessarily preclude a good diet. In fact, the right food choices can lead to a balanced meal even at such unlikely spots as the happy-hour buffet, the cocktail party, or the drive-through eatery.

Eating on the run is not the ideal way to nourish the body, but if you have to do it, do it with some thought. A little bit of planning can pay off with big nutritional benefits. The trick is to evaluate the available foods with an eye to their ingredients. Choose the snacks that contain complex carbohydrates, fibre, vitamins, and minerals, and protein sources without added fat. Granted, that's sometimes easier said than done, but with hosts and hostesses becoming more nutrition-conscious, it's a lot easier than it used to be.

Another trick is to satisfy your immediate hunger with healthy items, even when dining just on hors-d'oeuvres, so that the temptation to return for the rich snacks will be reduced. As a rule of thumb, avoid any item that's been deep fried.

The trendy term that's been applied to living off the hors-d'oeuvres tray is "grazing." Actually, the concept refers to many small feedings in a day as opposed to the traditional three big ones. There are, naturally, pros and cons to this approach to eating. Those in favour point to the fact that people who graze intelligently tend to accumulate less body fat than those who consume the same number of calories per day but all in one meal. The latter are uncharitably referred to as gorgers. The negative aspect is that grazers are liable to lose sight of the total picture and overdo one or two of the food groups — all fruit and veggies, or meat and cheese, that type of thing. Remember that variety, moderation, and balance are the keys, whether you're sitting down to three square meals a day, or grabbing a bite on the run.

Happy-Hour Buffet or Party: Enjoy fresh vegetables and fruit with yoghurt dips, whole grain breads and melba toast, low-fat spreads, lean meat, fish, or poultry. Check the recipes in the Appetizer section for more ideas. Avoid deep-fried foods, greasy snacks, and pastries.

At Home, No Time to Cook: Enjoy sandwiches made with whole-grain breads and lean meat, poultry, or fish, garnished with fresh vegetables; canned beans, toast, and salad; a bran muffin, yoghurt, and fruit; with fruit juice or milk for beverages. Avoid a dinner that consists of chips and pop. A meal doesn't have to be an elaborate affair involving hours in preparation, nor in fact does it have to be hot. The food groups can easily be represented in a sandwich — just don't fall into the fat trap of deep-fried snacks.

Skip Rope, Not Breakfast

One of the problems with giving the same bit of advice over and over again is that the listener eventually begins to tune out the message. This may be what happened to the recommendation to "start off each day with a good breakfast." People began to view it as one of those things that mothers always say, like "Be sure to look both ways" or "Don't hit your little brother'' — stuff you outgrow when you leave home.

But, wouldn't you know it, Mom was right again. Studies have shown over and over again that, no matter how you slice it, breakfast-skippers just don't perform as well physically or mentally. One of the landmark studies was conducted at the University of Iowa. Researchers used bicycle ergometers, treadmills, and maximum strength testers, and showed that physical ability was markedly decreased by late morning when breakfast was not eaten. Scholastic performance and attitude towards school work also deteriorated.

A study of 1,000 elementary school children in Lawrence, Massachusetts, supported the importance of breakfast as a positive influence on learning. A nutrition program for children from low-income families was started, and those children taking part in a school breakfast improved their test scores significantly more than students not in the program. Not only that, late arrival at school decreased, as did absenteeism.

And if improved mental and physical performance aren't enough, there's another bonus to starting the day with breakfast: you're more likely to get certain nutrients you miss out on at lunch and dinner. Breakfast-eaters are more likely to consume adequate amounts of vitamins C and D, riboflavin, and calcium than the skippers — and that's not even mentioning the fibre. It may be possible for a breakfast-skipper to have a bowl of whole grain cereal for lunch or dinner, but it's not very likely.

The Excuses

With all this going for it, why do you suppose so many people don't have breakfast? Three basic reasons are usually given: ''I'm not hungry,'' ''I don't have time,'' ''I'm on a diet.'' Not one of them holds water.

Let's look at ''I'm not hungry.'' Usually people who claim a lack of appetite in the morning are those who eat a light lunch, then really dig in for a late dinner. They often say that having breakfast actually makes them hungrier, which is probably true — for the short term. But the body can be retrained. After about two weeks of eating breakfast, the person will awaken with an appetite, and out-of-control hunger won't be a problem later in the day.

Those who cite ''no time'' as a reason for not eating breakfast are probably labouring under the misconception that breakfast has to be an elaborate hot meal, involving the stove and frying pan. Not so. Breakfast can be as quick as a blender shake, a bowl of cereal with fruit and milk, or a bran muffin, cheese, and apple. Setting the alarm clock 15 minutes earlier seems a small price to pay for improved energy and performance.

Finally, the biggest scam of all: ''I'm on a diet.'' Some people actually believe that, by omitting 300 or so calories at breakfast, they're making great strides in the battle of the bulge. The scale may show incontrovertible evidence to the contrary, and yet they still cling to the myth. In fact, the majority of people with a weight problem are breakfast-skippers. They usually compensate for the missed breakfast calories by snacking in the afternoon and by eating larger dinners. Perhaps it's time to harken back to the old saying: breakfast like a king, lunch like a prince, and dine like a pauper.

So then, how would a wise king break his fast? Well, some complex carbohydrates and fibre would be a good place to start. A bowl of cereal is a good choice. The cereal doesn't have to be hot, but if time permits there's nothing better on a snowy morning. There's a great variety of cold, ready-to-eat cereals available, many of which are excellent sources of fibre, vitamins and iron, and are low in fat. Whole wheat toast, pancakes or waffles with fruit, or hearty muffins with fruit and nuts are other tempting ways to jump-start your day. Browse through the recipe section for more ideas.

The protein part of breakfast can be the milk on your cereal or in your glass, some cheese with your muffin, cottage cheese on your toast, or a poached or boiled egg. Peanut butter on toast with banana is a popular item with kids. Light cream cheese on a whole wheat bagel might tempt some former breakfast-skippers, or they might go for yoghurt or cheese with applesauce on toast. The thing to avoid at breakfast is a rut.

That brings us to another important point: breakfast doesn't have to be breakfast. By which we mean that the traditional breakfast foods aren't the only ones that can be consumed as the sun peeks over the horizon. The important thing is to have foods that will give you a leg up on your day's requirement for vitamin C, complex carbohydrates, fibre, calcium, and some protein. Fruit salad and yoghurt; cold, leftover pizza with a whole wheat crust and low-fat toppings; split pea soup with some cheese, a muffin, and an orange juice chaser; brown rice with nuts and fruit. Okay, that last one's a little weird, but we're trying for a little adventure here.

If all of Canada woke up tomorrow morning and had a wholesome, nourishing breakfast, it would not solve our budget deficit, it wouldn't get agreement on nuclear disarmament, but we'd be one big step closer to a healthier society.

Brown-Bagging It, or,
Packing a Lunch That Packs a Nutritional Wallop
In simpler times jobs were nearer home, most of the fathers and children came home for the noon meal, and most of the people who prepared that meal were mothers. Okay, so times change, and we must keep up with the times. It's occasionally fun to have lunch in a restaurant (healthy choices can be made there), and it can be argued that big business deals just can't be negotiated over a peanut butter and banana sandwich. While brown-bagging it isn't everyone's idea of a noontime energizer, in actual fact the do-it-yourself lunch can be a lot easier on your health and on your wallet.

People who brown-bag their lunch can be divided into two groups: those with access to refrigeration and those without. For the first group, the choices for a good lunch are almost unlimited. The second group must focus their choices on foods that won't spoil in three or four hours. But a number of foods can be kept at room temperature and taste good, too.

The Earl of Sandwich was no dummy, and his wonderful innovation has been a boon to the lunch-box set for many years. The contents of the sandwich are limited only by the range of your imagination and your taste buds.

The Wrap Around

The cornerstone of the sandwich, of course, is bread, but that doesn't mean it has to be the sliced kind. There is no end of "breadstuffs" in which to place a filling. The smart sandwich maker will choose whole grain. Whole wheat bread, rye, pumpernickel, and whole wheat English muffins are but some of the choices available.

From the Middle East, we also have the wonderful pita bread, or pocket sandwich. Available at most supermarkets, this little pocket of bread can be stuffed with all your favourite sandwich fillings. Choose whole wheat pita if possible, for extra fibre.

The next item in the sandwich is the butter or margarine. Before automatically slapping it on, ask yourself why. Butter or margarine provide moisture and prevent the filling from seeping through the bread. But if you're going to put some mayonnaise on top of that, stop and use just one or the other. To control fat, use less of either or maybe choose one of the "lights." Better still, use other condiments—spicy mustards, relish, Mexican sauce, that type of thing. These contain less fat.

The Go Between

The protein part of your sandwich might follow the traditional choices of lean meat, poultry, fish, peanut butter, or cheese, but a little imagination in this department does wonders. How about cottage cheese and chopped pineapple; mashed beans with jalapeno peppers; salmon and light cream cheese with onions?

Vegetable additions are endless, from the usual tomato and lettuce to zucchini, cucumber, alfalfa sprouts, spinach, cabbage, onion, grated carrot, green pepper, mushrooms—you name it. And don't forget fruit as a sandwich ingredient as well. Bananas are a natural with peanut butter, but mashed or sliced peaches or pears, grated apple, or mandarin orange segments are a pleasant surprise with, for example, diced chicken.

Salads

Terrific as it is, giving us each day our daily sandwich can become dull and boring. From the wonderful world of plastic come great little containers in which to carry a variety of nutritious goodies. Foods from each of the food groups can satisfy the need for variety and adventure. A salad is an obvious choice and can be as imaginative as one you'd serve for dinner. Toss in some meat, eggs, or cheese cubes. Take along some whole wheat crackers, bread sticks, or a muffin—there's healthy eating! The trick with a portable salad is to bring the dressing in a separate container and add it just before eating.

Cold casseroles from last night's dinner can reappear at lunch-time, as can a cold pasta salad or brown rice dish. Some people even like cold pizza, especially if they made their own using low-fat toppings and cheese.

Block Bacteria from Your Bag

But what about those of us with no handy little refrigerator in the lunch room or even no lunch-room? The problem here is food preservation,

BROWN BAG CHOICES

Try to bag at least one food from each of the food groups: milk, meat, fruits and vegetables, breads and cereals.

Bread
whole wheat
rye
pumpernickel
english muffin
pita
bagel
muffins
bread sticks
melba toast

Filling
lean meat
lean poultry
salmon
tuna (water packed)
cheese
cottage cheese
light cream cheese
peanut butter
baked beans

Vegetables/Fruit
lettuce
spinach
zucchini
cucumber
tomato

alfalfa sprouts
cabbage
onion
celery
green pepper
grated carrot
grated apples
bananas
raisins
pineapple chunks
peaches
pears
mandarin orange segments

Salads
(*Check the recipe section for more ideas*)
tossed salad
bean salad
carrot and raisin salad
coleslaw
potato salad
pasta salad

Desserts
yoghurt
canned pudding
fresh fruit
fruit breads
cookies and squares

Thirst Quenchers
water
milk
fruit juice
vegetable juice
soups and broths

and the problem varies with the season. People who work out of doors are sometimes faced with food spoilage from the heat; other times a pickaxe may be needed to break into the frozen mass.

If lunch is to be kept indoors but not refrigerated, the freezer is a simple solution. Peanut butter and cheese sandwiches tolerate room temperature very well, but can be boring day after day. Some types of sandwiches can be frozen the night before. Take what you need from the freezer in the morning and they'll be thawed by noon. Sandwiches such as chicken or cold meat survive best in the freezer, but pack the lettuce and tomatoes separately. Small boxes of juices can also be frozen to serve as handy little ice packs. And they provide a cool drink with lunch. Use a thermos — the wide-necked variety is especially useful — for soups or drinks. The bottom line is keep hot foods hot and cold foods cold.

Just Desserts

For dessert there's always fresh fruit or canned items, like puddings, yoghurt, or fruit salad. Cake, donuts, and cookies are always tempting, but since they're often loaded with fat and calories, they aren't the best choice. To satisfy your desire for something sweet, you might bundle up a little packet of fruit-filled cereal squares, oatmeal bars, or carrot cake. Flip through the recipes in the Baked Goods section for some more ideas.

Milk and juices are handy beverages — you don't need a dietitian to tell you that they're more nutritious than a can of pop. Make sure you choose a fruit juice — not a fruit "drink."

Kids' Lunches

All these suggestions apply equally to children. Kids are pretty much like adults in that some of them want a lot of variety and some of them like the security of routine, familiar fare. It is best not to spring an eggplant sandwich on them without warning. For the most part, children's lunches are more acceptable (and are not tossed away or traded in the school yard) when the child has played a part in the planning and making of the lunch. They are less likely to throw away something they made themselves.

Eating well doesn't have to be boring, and you don't have to be a fanatic or a "nutrition nut" to realize that years of bad lunches can have a bad effect on your health. Packing a nutritious lunch can pack a healthy wallop in the future. If you're lucky (or unlucky, depending on your point of view) you'll spend about 40 years in the workforce, totalling up to 9,440 lunches. Plan ahead and you'll save money, be well nourished, and come out of it with more than a gold watch.

Healthy Snacking

While many purists would have people consume three perfect meals a day, we must come to grips with the fact that we don't live in a perfect world, and snacking isn't necessarily imperfect. In fact, when done properly, snacks can contribute important nutrients to the day's total intake.

Parents have many concerns about snacks: they contain empty calories, are bad for the teeth, ruin the appetite, and — the catchall concern — they're junk food. But not all food that's called junk food deserves the title. Let's take french fries as an example. Before you turn blue at the thought of fries as a part of healthy eating, let's analyze their good points and the bad. Bad news first. The major problem with fries is the quantity of fat they absorb in the cooking process. Two hundred grams of baked potato, your average spud, gives you a trace of fat. The same amount cooked in deep fat donates 32 grams to your fat bank. Potatoes lose a lot of their fibre once you peel them, but aside from that, both the baked and fried versions are sources of complex carbohydrates, potassium, vitamin C, niacin, and folic acid. If you buy frozen french fries and heat them in the oven, you cut the fat in half, but it's still a lot more than you'd get from a baked potato. But again, trying to put things into perspective, 200 grams of fries is a lot of fries. A typical serving would be less than half of this. Even the most dedicated fast-fooder is unlikely to pack away that much in one sitting.

All in all, then, french fries pack a fatty wallop, but they do contain some nutrients — so enjoy them, but only as an occasional treat.

What about the day-in and day-out kind of snacks that kids like? The problem with most of them — cookies, chips, chocolate bars — is too much fat. But there are alternatives. Take frozen dessert snacks. Sherbet has almost no fat; many frozen yoghurts have no more than 3 percent fat and lots of nutrients to boot. Old-fashioned popsicles have no fat, but precious few nutrients either. They are gradually being pushed out of the picture by frozen fruit juice bars on a stick. Try making your own Icy Yoghurt Pops using the recipe on page 213.

Fruit is always a good snack, but be careful of some of the new gussied-up versions. Fruit leather plays havoc with the teeth and banana chips have more to do with fat than bananas. Instead of cookies, kids will often go for crackers with an interesting spread. Try some of the low-fat variations in the recipe section. Breadsticks or pretzels, especially if you buy the unsalted kind, are a fun snack with barely a trace of fat. And don't forget cereals as a snack as well — not just the sitdown bowl of cereal with milk variety, but a little bundle eaten from the hand. Good snackin'!

Finally — and this is meant mostly for adults since kids might be a little resistant — don't forget dried fruit, like figs and dates and apricots. Whole or chopped up and mixed with some slivered almonds, this is a snack that anyone would love. Remember to brush after, since dried fruit can be a problem for teeth, because it sticks to them and provides a breeding ground for bacteria.

Snacking doesn't have to be a bad thing — it just takes a little thought to turn it into a good thing.

Healthy Eating on a Budget

There's no getting around it — for many people times are tough. It's enough to break your bank-book and your heart. A concern of dietitians these days is that in an effort to save money on the grocery bill, people may be choosing low-cost, high-fat foods on which to fill up. It is pos-

Photos: Pesto Spread, page 45, and Oriental Crab Spread, page 51 (facing page)
Babsi's Broccoli Soup, page 59 (overleaf)

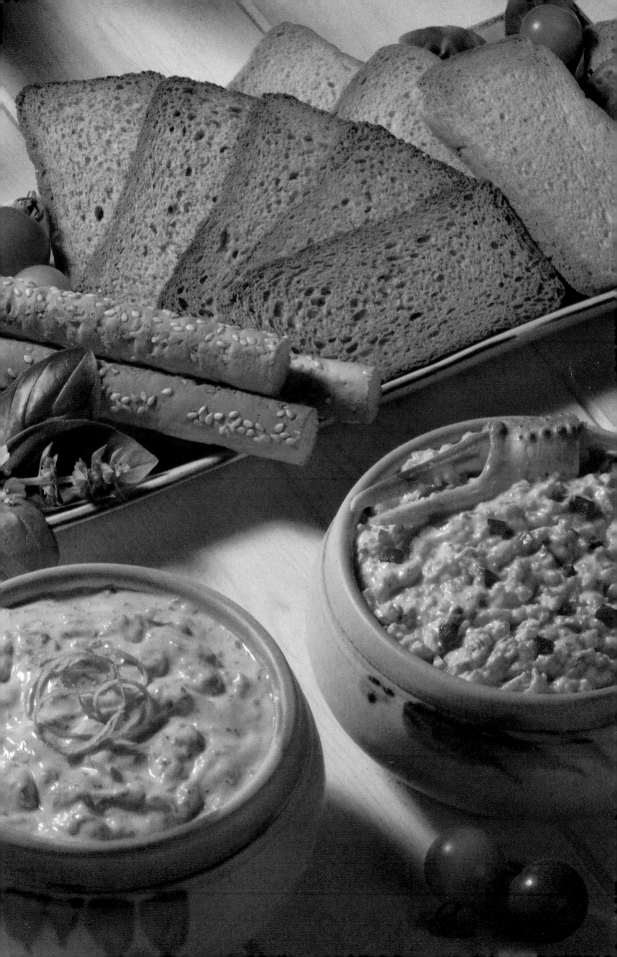

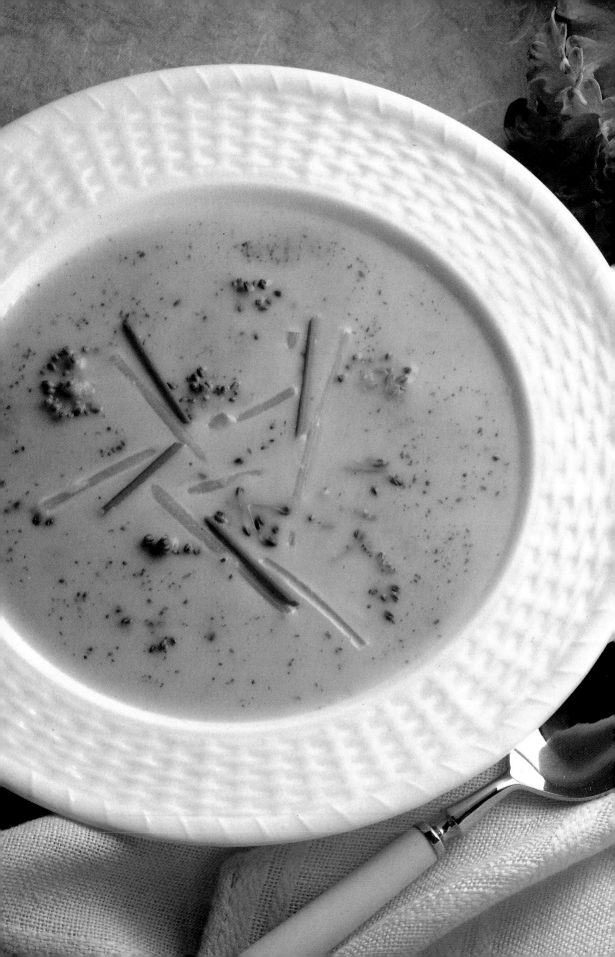

sible to shop economically and still select healthful foods. Some of the tips that follow may well be ones you learned at your mother's knee, but got out of the habit of using. Some may be new to you. We hope they will help you meet the challenge of getting absolutely the most nutrients from your dollars.

General Tips

Base your weekly menu planning on Canada's Food Guide. The next time you shop, list the foods you buy opposite the food groups in which they belong; you'll be sure your family is getting a well-balanced menu.

Plan your menus a week at a time, and, if possible, shop only once a week. By looking ahead, you can plan for leftovers and make use of what you already have on hand.

Check the newspaper and grocery store ads for weekly specials and sales. They'll help you plan your menus according to the best buys. Wednesday night is a good time to do your menu planning since most of the store specials are in Wednesday's paper.

If you have some extra money, buy large quantities of staple items (canned goods, cereals, rice, pasta, etc.) if they are a really good deal. If you have a freezer, take advantage of sales.

Stick to your shopping list, but if you find a better buy, go for it. Flexibility is a key factor.

Make friends with generic or store brands. While not the fancy quality (the peas may not all be the same size, for example), these are usually good buys of acceptable quality.

Compare costs for the same food in the fresh, frozen, and canned sections of your supermarket. Which is the best to buy? To find out, divide the price by the number of servings you get. The lower price per serving is your best buy, whether it's fresh, frozen, or canned. From a nutritional standpoint, the canned product usually contains more sodium or sugar, but a quick rinse under the tap can help that.

This is an old one, but still valid. Eat before you shop. If you go to the store hungry, your shopping list doesn't stand a chance.

Never economize on nutrition. Shop for foods that are good sources of the important nutrients. Buy as many of these as your budget allows, with the greatest possible variety.

Take advantage of unit pricing for comparison shopping. Granted, sometimes you have to be a contortionist to read the little labels, but they are a good tool for budget watching.

Nowadays, when convenience has become an almost essential commodity, one shouldn't abandon all timesavers; some convenience foods, like bread, cost less than the ''made-from-scratch'' variety. Check products carefully to see how much time you're saving at what price. Pancake mixes are an example of money spent for not that much time saved.

Bulk foods are almost always a savings—but note the "almost." Spices and herbs cost more when fancy bottles are used and the premixed combinations should be avoided. It's no big deal to mix your own cinnamon and sugar, but you pay through the nose when a company does it for you. Keep your own mixes in properly sealed jars to preserve flavour and aroma.

Keep two jars in the refrigerator, one marked "vegetable" and the other "fruit." Into the former, pour liquids from cooking and canned vegetables for use in soups and stews. In the latter go juices from canned fruit that can be used with plain gelatin to make your own jelly desserts.

Fruits and Vegetables
When buying greens, don't automatically assume that lettuce is the best buy for your nutritional dollar, just because it's cheaper. Other types of greens may be more nutritious and sometimes cost the same or less per kilogram.

Precut cabbage or coleslaw mixture is a bad idea: having somebody else chop it for you loses nutrients and adds cost. Ditto for frozen vegetables in sauce. It doesn't take long to make your own sauce — plus you can control the amount of fat in it.

Large bags of frozen vegetables are a better buy than the little packages, and you need cook only as much as required. Be careful to reseal the package tightly to prevent the remainder from drying out.

Cook vegetables with as little water and for as short a time as necessary to make them palatable, in order to save vitamins and minerals. A steamer, microwave, or pressure cooker is helpful here.

If bananas become overripe, don't assign them to the garbage can, put them in the freezer. They'll turn black, all right, but they'll be great for banana bread, muffins, and so on.

Dairy Products
When buying milk products, consider lower fat varieties, and bear in mind that the milk products group is about the most nutrient-dense — more nutrients, less money.

For cooking and baking, use powdered skim milk; for drinking, if your family isn't thrilled with the reconstituted stuff, try mixing it with fresh milk. It tastes better if you make it the day before. Serve it from the fresh milk container.

Try to avoid a knee-jerk reaction to the term "processed" as applied to cheese. You still get protein, calcium, riboflavin, and other nutrients from the processed spreads and slices, but the price is lower. The one drawback is the additional sodium.

Leftover cheese can be frozen for later use in casseroles, lasagna, and so on. Only its texture changes, making it a little too crumbly to thaw out and serve as cheese pieces.

If you own a yoghurt maker, make use of it. Almost any recipe that calls for sour cream will accept yoghurt instead, with a great nutritional pay-off. Actually, you don't even need a yoghurt maker to make your own. Check out the recipe in the dessert section (page 226) for instructions.

Cottage cheese is a great addition to many recipes, and a great source of calcium and protein. It freezes well, so if you think you won't have a chance to use it before it goes bad, pop it in the freezer.

Breads and Cereals

Whether as a breakfast food, an addition to meat loaf, or part of a fruit cobbler, cereal is a great source of low-cost nutrition. But, again, compare the cost of plain cereals with that of those with added dried fruit and sugar.

Day-old baked breads, rolls, and muffins are usually marked down but are still as fresh as if you'd bought them yesterday and stored them at home. If you have enough freezer space, buy enough of these marked-down goods for a week at a time.

Save the end slices of bread and those that are too dry for ordinary use. Crushed and crumbled, they make great toppings for casseroles; coatings or stuffings for meats, poultry, or fish.

Pasta, rice, and cereal are other great meat stretchers. They combine well with so many flavours that an almost endless variety of dinners is possible when you use them. Add a glass of milk or a piece of cheese, bread, and carrot sticks and you've got a meal that will satisfy the heftiest appetite and smallest budget.

The best buy in rice, in terms of nutrients for your dollar, is definitely brown. The taste is "nutty" and lends itself to many interesting recipes. If brown isn't your cup of tea, go for long-grain converted, then plain white. The instant or quick rices are the most expensive.

Eggs

Along with milk, eggs give you the most nutrients per dollar. They're a real bargain, especially for their high-quality protein. Just don't cook them in added fat. The one thing to watch with eggs are their cholesterol content and, as with liver, that only applies if your cholesterol handling mechanism is out of whack (that is, you have elevated blood cholesterol levels). Egg whites contain no cholesterol.

When comparing the prices of eggs of different sizes, keep this formula in mind: if the difference in price per dozen between the medium and large egg is seven cents or more, the medium size is the better buy. If the difference is six cents or less, buy the large size.

Meat and Fish

Tightening up on your budget doesn't mean you should eliminate meat. You'll lose many important and essential nutrients in the bargain. Take a glance at Canada's Food Guide. You'll see that the suggested servings of meat are not large.

If meat is on the menu, use the cost per serving, not the cost per kilogram, as your guide. For example, a boneless pot roast may cost more per kilo than one with the bone in, but because there's less waste, each serving will cost less. Remember the following guideline: a half-kilogram (one pound) of boneless meat will serve four; the same amount with a bone in will serve two. If it's really bony, like spare ribs, you'll need a half-kilogram per person.

Use the old extender trick. A smaller portion of meat served with pasta, rice, cheese, eggs, beans, and vegetables will give a lot more nutritional mileage and that, of course, is why we have casseroles and stir-fry.

Nothing will save you more meat money than cooking at a lower temperature — never higher than 300°F. Some experts even recommend 275°F. Meats cooked at low temperatures not only shrink less, but are more tender and have more flavour than those cooked at high temperatures.

When buying foods for lunch boxes, compare the cost of presliced and packaged cold cuts to those sold in a solid piece. You generally pay more if the meat packing company does the slicing and packaging.

Think ''tenderizer'' — either the natural chemical kind (papain) or the kind you provide with a wooden or metal meat mallet. Tough cuts are just as nutritious as the more expensive, and often have less fat. You just need to treat 'em rough. Marinating the night before is a good idea as well. Check the recipes in the Main Course section for some tasty marinade ideas.

For steak on a budget, choose chuck, bottom round, or ''shoulder'' steak. Marinate or tenderize it first, then broil or grill to medium rare for maximum tenderness.

Meat counters carry ready-cubed beef for stewing. But because store labour and meat trimmings cost money, you'll rate a double dividend if you buy beef chuck and cut it yourself. Then simmer the bone and trimmings for broth to make soup.

When buying poultry, remember that the larger the bird, the greater the ratio of meat to bone. Bear in mind, also, that since it takes so little additional time and fuel to roast a larger bird, it's smart to buy a big one that will give you extra for snacks or a second dinner.

When cooking turkey or chicken, take the wing tips, back, heart, neck, and gizzard — any parts your family may not care to eat — and freeze them. When additional spare parts accumulate, make your own broth (see page 52).

Utility-grade poultry does not mean a bird is only fit for a labour camp. It's just one that met with an accident between the coop and the counter. Maybe it has a missing wing tip, or a skinned breast — nothing major. Utility is usually your best buy for chicken and turkey.

The cost of fresh fish varies depending on the time of year. Start thinking in terms of 100 grams. It's easy—100 grams serves one person if you're buying fillets.

Frozen fish fillets can be a really good buy, considering there's absolutely no waste.

Canned fish, usually tuna or salmon, is great for any number of dishes. Families may have preferences, but, generally speaking, cheaper is better. As an example, light flaked tuna may not look as good as fancy white, but it's every bit as nutritious and a whole lot less expensive. Water- or broth-packed is a good choice.

One can't overstate the value of sardines as an inexpensive source of nutrition—protein, calcium, vitamins, you name it. You can even find them packed in fat-free sauces like tomato and mustard.

As an alternative to meat, you can't do better than beans. Canned beans are acceptable if time is too short to make your own, but large batches can be baked and frozen for later use.

Know your beans. Learn to use different kinds: white beans, kidney beans, garbanzos, split peas, lentils—the list goes on. They're rich in protein, fibre, and nutrients, and they're inexpensive.

The following is an example of a nutritional label that shows a breakdown for a type of bread.

NUTRITION INFORMATION per 76 g serving (2 slices)		
Energy	190	Cal
	790	kJ
Protein	6.7	g
Fat	4.5	g
Polyunsaturates	0.9	g
Monounsaturates	1.6	g
Saturates	0.9	g
Cholesterol	0	mg
Carbohydrate	33.6	g
Dietary fibre	2.7	g
Sodium	358	mg
Potassium	112	mg

Percentage of Recommended Daily Intake	
	%
Thiamin	20
Riboflavin	6
Niacin	8
Folacin	5
Calcium	2
Phosphorus	11
Magnesium	16
Iron	20
Zinc	9

Ingredients: Unbleached enriched flour, water, oat bran, oatmeal, glucose, fructose, or sugar, vegetable oil shortening, fancy molasses, salt, raisin juice concentrate, wheat gluten, yeast*, sodium stearoyl-2-lactylate, mono and diglycerides, contains a topping of rolled oats.
*order may change.

Nutrition Labelling

In response to the growing demand from Canadians for more information regarding the nutritional value of the food they buy, new nutrition labelling guidelines have been created. To help you achieve routine healthy eating, the federal government, consumer groups, the food industry, dietitians and other health specialists combined efforts to help the Canadian consumer take advantage of nutrition information when making food choices in the supermarket. While food manufacturers aren't required by law to provide nutrition information, those who do so have strict guidelines concerning the information on the label. If a claim is made about the nutrient content of a particular item, the manufacturer must provide evidence that the claims are true.

Take fat as an example. For a long time now we've seen labels like "fat reduced," "low fat," and "light." But what did they really mean? Now, if a label says "low fat" the manufacturer will have to tell you just how much fat there is. Furthermore, if the type of fat is stated, then the new regulations require you be given the amounts of the three major types of fat: polyunsaturates, monounsaturates, saturates, plus the amount of cholesterol in the food.

Similarly, if the label makes reference to carbohydrate content, you'll see a breakdown of the amounts of sugar, starch and fibre. If sodium is mentioned, then you'll also be given the potassium content giving a balanced view, so to speak.

The basic information on any nutrition label is that which is called the "core" list. This will present the amount of carbohydrate, fat and protein in an average serving of the food product, along with the calorie or energy content. Metric buffs will be happy to know that energy will also be presented in kilojoules.

Regulations have been made regarding vitamins and minerals as well. Before these nutrients are presented under the headings "contains" or "source of," they must provide at least five percent of the Recommended Daily Intake. If they're said to be "high" or a "good source" then 15 percent of the RDI must be present and in order to rate a "very high" or "excellent source" the vitamin or mineral must be present in an amount that is at least 25 percent of the RDI, 50 percent if the claim is being made for vitamin C.

Claims for fibre are being controlled as well. In order to qualify as a "very high source" of fibre, the labelled food product must contain at least six grams of fibre per serving. Four grams rates a "high source" and two grams allows it to boast itself as a "source" of dietary fibre.

It will help you to deal better with the term "low fat" if you understand that the new regulations determine that a food making that claim cannot have more than three grams of fat per serving and not more than 15 percent of the "dry matter" (excluding moisture) can be fat. The term "low saturates" means you'll get no more than two grams of saturated fats in a serving of the food and not more than 15 percent of the calories in that food come from saturates. If "low cholesterol" is a product's boast, then it must give you no more than 20 milligrams of cholesterol

Don't be frightened off by the word "processed." Processing simply means a food has been altered in some way to make it safer, easier to use and have a longer shelf life. Processing also means we have a wide variety of foods available to us all year long. In many cases the alteration is not great enough to threaten the food's nutritional status and, if we're being realistic, we must accept that for busy lives convenience is an important factor. Macaroni and cheese is probably a good example. Yes, it would be great to make your own pasta and use a chunk of natural cheese. But the kind that comes in a box is quick, the kids love it and it does provide B vitamins, iron, protein, and calcium. Serve it with whole wheat bread, salad, a glass of milk, and fresh fruit for dessert — everybody's happy.

in a serving or in 100 grams (about 3 oz.) of the food and be low in saturated fats as well.

A food declaring itself "cholesterol free" is allowed to have no more than three milligrams of cholesterol per 100 grams and, again, must be low in saturated fatty acids. An example of how this works could be found on the label of a box of vegetable shortening. While it in fact contains no dietary cholesterol, it won't be able to make that claim since it does exceed the maximum of saturated fats stipulated in the regulations.

Nutrition labelling isn't the solution to all our nutrition problems, a lot of educating still needs to be done but it's definitely a step in the right direction.

The Nutritional Feeding of Your Mind

It never let's up, does it? Ever since you were a kid, somebody's been nagging you about what goes into your mouth. First your mother, then your teacher, then your spouse. And if that's not enough, your own kids (being nutritionally aware as kids are nowadays) have to get in on the act. "Don't eat this, it's loaded with salt." "Don't eat that, it's got preservatives in it." "Don't eat the other thing, it's full of fat and not only that, if you like it, it must be bad for you!"

But where do people learn these nutritional tidbits they're so anxious to share with you? More to the point, where do you get your information about nutrition? Some people might ask a doctor or nurse about nutrition or, if they're in hospital, they might have the opportunity to talk to a dietitian. The popular press — books, magazines, newspapers devote increasing space to the topic of nutrition. Self-styled "nutritionists" offer counselling on the subject — often with no training or with a question-able degree from a non-accredited school or "university." Nutrition books are written by people with the initials Ph.D. and an unsuspecting public most often has no way of knowing whether the degree is valid. There are those who boast of being a "certified clinical nutritionist." Certified by whom? Promoters of nutrition nonsense can band together and give themselves a prestigious name. Unfortunately, they don't always have the educational background that would render their advice reliable. Laws governing freedom of speech permit these people to say anything that strikes their fancy, regardless of accuracy. And there is no law protecting the term "nutritionist" — anyone can claim to be one. However, there are laws regarding use of the term "Registered Dieti-tian." (The initials R.D. after someone's name means Registered Die-titian. These initials can vary from province to province, so look for any of R.P.Dt., P.Dt., R.D., R.Dt., or R.D.N. The French version is dt.p.) These initials will tell you that the dietitian has graduated with a degree in nutrition from an accredited university and has fulfilled the require-ments for membership in the Dietetic Association.

A dietitian first earns a four year Bachelor's degree Bachelor of Sci-ence in Nutrition, Bachelor of Home Economics, Bachelor of Human

Ecology, depending on the university he or she attends. The important thing is that it is an "accredited" program in an "accredited" university, which means that the program and university have been sanctioned by an educational body established to verify their authenticity. In other words, someone has to check to see that those teaching the course are qualified to do so. Then The Canadian Dietetic Association reviews dietetic programs to make sure they meet approved standards.

During the four years, the dietetic student studies, among other subjects, chemistry, biochemistry, biology, physiology, food science, and, of course, nutrition. As well as attaining the knowledge through the Bachelor's degree, a program of practical experience is also required to demonstrate that the student can apply the knowledge gained. Dietitians may also opt to pursue a master's degree or doctorate.

Dietitians are the professionals that have the skills and expertise to translate scientific nutrition research into practical dietary advice for consumers. Dietitians apply their knowledge and skills in nutrition for everyday living (e.g., pregnancy, infant feeding, fitness), and in developing therapeutic diets and planning meals for large groups and institutions. Dietitians work in a wide variety of areas. They are found in traditional health care settings such as hospitals and other institutions, government health departments and outpatient clinics. They are also found in business settings such as the food industry, food service industry and food marketing boards. Many work in academic institutions, private practice, research, media, and consumer information services.

When looking for nutrition information, check out the qualifications of your source. You take your car to a licensed mechanic, you have your hair done by a licensed beautician. Be at least as fair to your body.

If you have questions on nutrition, contact dietitians in hospitals, government departments (such as the department of health), in industry, or in private practice. Your local dietetic association can direct you to a qualified dietitian.

Alberta Registered Dietitians Association
370 Terrace Plaza
4445 Calgary Trail South
Edmonton, Alberta
T6H 5R7

British Columbia Dietitians' and Nutritionists' Association
1037 West Broadway, Suite 306
Vancouver, British Columbia
V6H 1E3

Corporation professionelle des diététistes du Quebec
4205 rue St. Denis, bureau 250
Montreal, Quebec
H2J 2K9

Manitoba Association of Registered Dietitians
320 Sherbrook Street
Winnipeg, Manitoba
R3B 2W6

New Brunswick Association of Dietitians
P.O. Box 4102
Moncton, New Brunswick
E1A 6E7

Newfoundland Dietetic Association
P.O. Box 1756
St. John's, Newfoundland
A1C 5P5

Northern Nutrition Association
Box 116
Yellowknife, Northwest Territories
X1A 2N1

Nova Scotia Dietetic Association
Box 8841, Station A
Halifax, Nova Scotia
B3K 5M5

Ontario Dietetic Association
480 University Avenue, Suite 601
Toronto, Ontario
M5G 1V2

Prince Edward Island Dietetic Association
P.O. Box 2575
Charlottetown, Prince Edward Island
C1A 8C2

Saskatchewan Dietetic Association
845 Broad Street
Box 390
Regina, Saskatchewan
S4P 3G7

Part Two | PUTTING IT ALL TOGETHER

We hope that as you scan the recipes in this book, you'll find yourself wanting to try one recipe after another. But remember, each recipe is nothing more than instructions for one dish, one small part of what is needed for a complete meal. Recipes seldom stand on their own. They are just part of a larger nutritional plan—the plan for one meal, a day's meals, maybe even a week's meals.

Meal planning gives you the chance to put it all together, all the nutritional information, all the recipes, all the groceries you buy each week — into a practical approach to good nutrition. Although it may sound difficult, meal planning is not hard to do. It takes some common sense, a good eye, a little practice, and, sometimes, a bit of quick addition in your head.

The purpose of planning meals is to make sure you get your fair share of nutrients and dietary fibre, while keeping calories and fat and other nutrients within healthy levels. It's the sum of what you eat that matters, not the individual foods. By balancing different foods, you'll come out at the end of the day nutritionally on target.

Whether you're making or buying a meal, keep our four nutrition guidelines in mind.

1. VARIETY
Does the meal have at least three or four different kinds of food in it? By eating a variety of foods, you have the best assurance that you are getting all the nutrients you need. Variety means not only choosing foods from all the food groups, but also choosing different foods from any one food group. Eat different foods every day, and you will be sure of getting variety in your diet.

2. FAT
Where is the fat coming from in the meal? Fat adds staying power, so you want to have some fat at every meal, but you don't want to overdo it. Just remember to make up for a high-fat dish by eating other lower-fat foods in the same meal and throughout the rest of the day.

To help you, remember that only 30 percent of the calories should come from fat. Therefore, a woman should aim to keep her fat intake to about 65 grams each day. A man would be limited to about 90 grams of fat a day.*

*Thirty percent of 1900 is 570 calories. To convert calories to grams of fat, divide 570 by 9, because there are 9 calories in every gram of fat. (30 percent of 2700 = 810; 810 divided by 9 = 90).

3. COMPLEX CARBOHYDRATES AND FIBRE
Does the meal contain a source of complex carbohydrates (such as bread,

cereal, fruit, vegetables, or legumes)? How many fibre-rich foods are in the meal? Fibre helps to make a meal more satisfying by filling you up without too much fat. Not every food has to be filled with fibre. It's quite all right to eat low-fibre French bread—as long as your needs for dietary fibre are being met in other foods.

Canadians currently eat about 15 grams of fibre a day. It is recommended that we should try to double this amount to approximately 30 grams of fibre a day.

4. CALORIES

Maintaining a healthy weight means balancing calories consumed as food with those burned off in activity. The average woman between the ages of 25 and 49 needs about 1,900 calories a day. An average man of the same age needs about 2,700 calories. If you're younger or more active, you'll need more calories, and if you're older or not very active, you'll need fewer calories.

This is what meal planning is all about. It's a juggling act, balancing the positives and the negatives to come out with a nutritious end product.

Although you might not go through the day with calculator in hand, the nutrient values given for the recipes in this book will help you judge each recipe and how it influences the value of the whole meal. In time, you will be able to assess a recipe and a meal by the ingredients it contains. Then, using this information, you can decide about what else you are going to eat, so that you end your day on target nutritionally.

DAILY NUTRITION GUIDELINES

	Women (25-49 yrs.)	*Men (25-49 yrs.)*
Calories	1900	2700
Fat	65 grams	90 grams
Fibre	30 grams	30 grams

One Consumer's Meal for a Day

Let's take as an example a day's menu for a thirty-year-old woman. Recipes included in this book are marked with an asterisk.

Breakfast
- ½ grapefruit
- 1 cup/250 mL bran flakes
- ½ cup/125 mL 2 percent milk
- coffee with ¼ cup/50 mL 2 percent milk

Hot or ready-to-eat, cereal is a good choice for a low-fat start to the day. The bran cereal and fresh fruit make this a fibre-packed meal. At a glance you can see that this meal is low in fat, leaving some flexibility for planning lunch and dinner. The variety of foods is also good, with three food groups represented.

Morning Break
- 1 Cranberry Oat Muffin*
- coffee with ¼ cup/50 mL 2 percent milk

This muffin is a little higher in fat than some muffins, but since breakfast was low in fat, this choice is a reasonable one on this particular day. Muffins containing oat or wheat bran and dried fruits would give even more fibre.

Lunch
- bowl of Beef Barley Soup*
- 1 Whole Wheat Biscuit*
- 2 tsp./10 mL butter or margarine
- carrot and celery sticks
- 1 cup/250 mL 2 percent milk
- ½ cantaloupe

This meal, too, is an excellent source of dietary fibre because of the barley and vegetables in the soup, the whole wheat biscuit, the vegetable sticks, and the fruit. The major source of fat is the butter or margarine, which is fine in this meal because the other foods are quite low in fat. This woman might have skipped the butter or margarine had the main course been higher in fat or had a rich dessert been planned. So far, she has a good intake of fibre and a moderate amount of fat. There is some leeway left for planning dinner.

Afternoon Break
- 1 apple

Fruit is low-calorie, has no fat, and adds to the day's fibre intake.

Dinner
- Chicken and Broccoli Bake*
- Green Garden Salad with Sesame Vinaigrette*
- Geraldine's Cake*
- tea with 1 tsp./5 mL sugar and ¼ cup/50 mL milk

The day's meals are completed with a higher-fat dinner. Since the fibre intake for the day was well on track, and because fat has been kept in control during the rest of the day, the fat in the main course and the dessert are not a problem. Had this woman chosen a lower-fat main course, it might have been possible to eat something like Cheese and Herb Bread,* which is higher in fat than the whole wheat biscuit eaten at lunch.

At the day's end, this woman can be proud of how she combined her foods in keeping with the nutritional guidelines.

NUTRITIONAL VALUE OF THE DAY'S MEALS COMPARED TO THE GUIDELINES

Meal	Calories	Fat (grams)	Fibre (grams)
Breakfast	252	4.2	7.4
Morning snack	259	9.8	1.4
Lunch	587	18.9	11.0
Afternoon snack	80	—	3.5
Dinner	719	29.7	7.7
Total	**1897**	**62.6**	**31.0**
Guidelines	**1900**	**65.0**	**30.0**

Special Meals

Although it is the sum of the day's meals that really counts, some people find it useful to organize their day and their requirements by dividing them in thirds: morning, afternoon, and evening. Whether you eat three regular meals or six mini-meals a day, you can still plan your day in thirds. For example, the nutrients in breakfast and morning coffee break should be added together as the first third of your day.

For the average woman, a third of her nutrients would be about 650 calories, 22 grams of fat, and about 10 grams of fibre. This is the amount she could eat in each third of her day. Of course, there will be days on which she will eat light in the morning and afternoon, knowing that she is going out for dinner. Or she might have a big breakfast on the weekend and cut back on what she eats for the rest of the day.

To give you an idea of how to juggle your meals in the interest of good nutrition, take a look at these three different situations.

A Meal for Guests
Company is coming and you want to serve a special meal. You're dying to offer a decadent dessert, but you're a bit concerned about the calories and fat. What do you do? You simply plan for a small and low-fat main course, ensuring that your guests have room for the delicious dessert.

Menu
- Grape and Orange Sole Supreme*
- ½ cup/125 mL of fettucine
- Garden Green Salad with Raspberry Basil Vinaigrette*
- Deluxe Peas*
- Fluffy Pumpkin Cheesecake*
- coffee or tea

Nutritional Analysis

	Calories	Fat	Fibre
In the meal	672	23.9	8.2
Third of guidelines	650	22.0	10.0

A Meatless Meal

There are two ways to plan a meatless meal. If you choose a legume-and vegetable-based main course that is low in fat and high in fibre, you can afford a richer appetizer or dessert. But if you build your meal around cheese and eggs, which are higher in fat, you should look for lower-fat and higher-fibre foods such as whole grain bread, fruits, and vegetables, to go with the main course.

In the following menu, the low-fat spaghetti is balanced by the richer cheese and herb bread.

Menu
- spaghetti with Lentil Spaghetti Sauce*
- Cheese and Herb Bread*
- Spinach Salad with Creamy Garlic Dressing*
- 1 cup/250 mL 2 percent milk

Nutritional Analysis

	Calories	Fat	Fibre
In the meal	697	21.1	11.4
Third of guidelines	650	22.0	10.0

A Brown-Bag Lunch

Sandwiches, the stand-by for bag lunches, can pack away the fat. Typical luncheon meats, cheese, peanut butter, even salmon, can contribute significantly to your fat intake for the day. Try to balance the fat in your sandwich with high-fibre, low-fat whole grain bread, fresh vegetables, and fruit.

Menu
- salmon sandwich on whole wheat bread with lettuce and tomato and 1 tbsp./15 mL salad dressing
- orange
- 1 Carrot Bran Muffin*
- 1 cup/250 mL carton of skim milk

Nutritional Analysis

	Calories	Fat	Fibre
In the meal	650	19.7	10.9
Third of guidelines	650	22.0	10.0

As you can see, menu planning isn't really all that difficult. You don't have to be a dietitian to make sensible choices. And remember that all the recipes in this book have a nutritional analysis to help you make those choices. Enjoy experimenting with the recipes, and here's to healthy eating!

Note about Nutritional Analyses

All recipes were analysed using Imperial measures. Optional items and garnishes were not included in the nutrient analyses. Unless otherwise stated, the recipes were tested and analysed using 2 percent milk, 2 percent yoghurt, and 2 percent cottage cheese. If a range of servings is given, the analysis was done using the larger amount.

Microwave recipes were tested in a 600-700-watt, full-sized microwave oven. If your oven wattage is different, you may have to adjust cooking times. For microwave ovens without a turntable, rotating dishes once or twice during cooking is recommended for even cooking. Refer to the manufacturer's directions for your microwave oven if you need more information.

Note about Menu Suggestions

Most of the recipes are followed by menu suggestions developed by dietitians across Canada. These menu suggestions have been developed using the nutritional guidelines to illustrate how the recipes may be incorporated into a meal that meets the guidelines for variety, fat, and fibre.

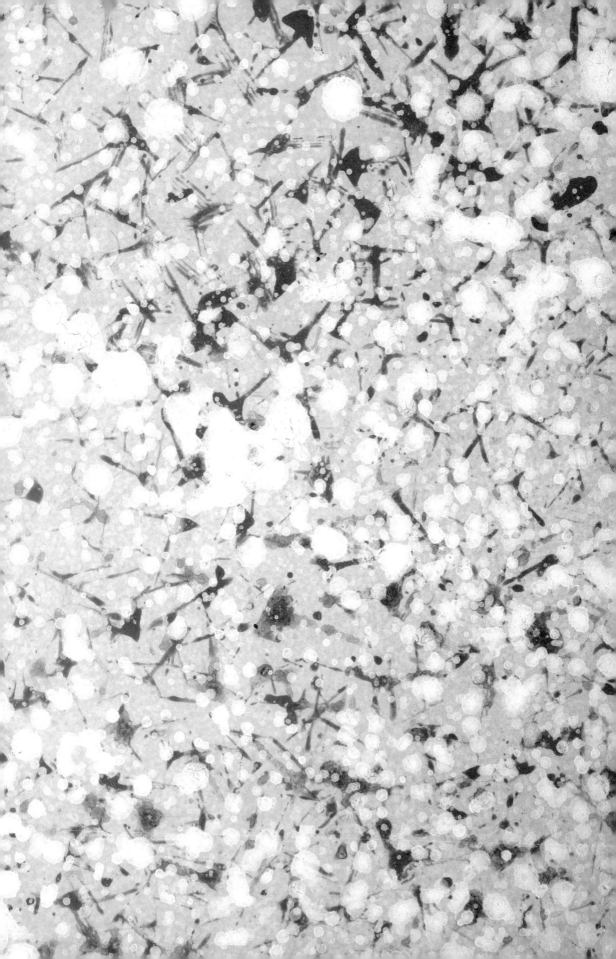

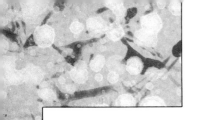

THE • EXCITING • VARIETY • OF

APPETIZERS

*Appetizing morsels of food are always in order, whether for
a reception, a cocktail party, an informal get-together,
an open house, or a small, intimate dinner party.
Add a combination of fine food, some friendly
people, and your own very special welcome,
and you have the ingredients for a
special event. The important
thing is to enjoy
your guests.*

The best appetizers are light enough to leave some room for the main course to follow, and easy enough to leave the cook time to enjoy the conversation. Appetizers should spark or tantalize the appetite, not dull it, and they should set the tone for the meal to follow. Formal get-togethers require a more sophisticated approach, like Eggplant Tapas (page 46) or Oriental Pork Rolls with Sweet and Sour Sauce (page 54); informal backyard barbecues call for fun starters, like Hot Veggies and Garlic Dip (page 50).

All your favourites are here — from dips and spreads to ethnic foods — and they're all lighter, easier, and lower in fat and calories, in keeping with today's life-styles. And some, like Whole-wheat Vegetarian Pizza (page 42) are great for munching, too.

Try Ingeleoge Vis (page 47) for an unusual and exciting presentation of fish fillets; or for a zippy prelude, try Lemon Pesto Spread (page 45) for melba toast, or Marinated Vegetables (page 48). This superb treatment for raw vegetables is a pleasant change from using them as crudités for dipping. Another favourite for years has been the popular Spinach Dip (page 52) prepared with a commercial vegetable soup mix and sour cream and served in a hollowed-out loaf of rye or pumpernickel bread. Try our new ''lighter'' made-from-scratch version, which is much lower in fat and sodium but equally as delicious.

You can serve one or two appetizers before a meal or build a whole meal around several of them. Smaller portions of several appetizers, chosen carefully with nutrition and Canada's Food Guide in mind, can become a complete meal. Select different flavours, different temperatures (some hot, some refrigerated), and different textures. Put enough of these together, and you'll have a light luncheon or dinner that covers all of the food groups.

''LITTLE MEAL'' MENU
Hummus with raw vegetable dippers and pita triangles (page 53)
Spinach Dip (page 52)
Oriental Pork Rolls (page 54)
Pineapple Fruit Plate with Dip (page 225)
*(this can be an appetizer or dessert depending
on the rest of the menu)*

Tips for Dips

Mexican salsa combined with plain low-fat yoghurt is a quickly
prepared dip for raw vegetables or unsalted tortilla chips.
Another easily prepared dip with a Mexican fiesta flavour: to
plain yoghurt, add chili powder and garlic powder to taste.

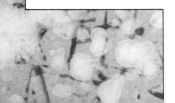

Besides the price, what's the difference between red and green peppers? Green peppers are just immature red ones. If left to ripen, green peppers turn red and become sweeter. Red or green, one medium-sized pepper provides about 35 calories and is an excellent source of vitamin C.

WHOLE WHEAT VEGETARIAN PIZZA
Susie Sziklai, Vancouver, British Columbia

Offer these pizzas as a healthy snack for pre-dinner or evening munching. They can also be the focal point for a tasty lunch. Vary the vegetable toppings by using some of the new coloured peppers showing up in the stores — orange, yellow, and purple.

6	whole wheat pita breads	6
1	can (7.5 oz./213 mL) tomato sauce	1
2 tbsp.	Italian seasoning	25 mL
15	mushrooms, thinly sliced	15
1	green pepper, cut into strips	1
1	small onion, coarsely chopped	1
2 cups	shredded mozzarella cheese	500 mL
½ cup	shredded feta cheese	125 mL
1 tbsp.	dried oregano	15 mL

Flatten pitas; spread with a layer of tomato sauce; sprinkle with Italian seasoning. Top with mushrooms, green pepper, onion, and cheese. Sprinkle with oregano. Place on ungreased baking sheet. Bake in 400°F (200°C) oven for about 10 minutes. Cut into triangles with kitchen scissors.

MENU SUGGESTION
These crunchy pizzas contribute calcium and dietary fibre. Skim-milk mozzarella can be used to decrease the amount of fat in the recipe. Add a milk-based chowder (rich in calcium), a tossed salad with oil-free dressing, and a fresh fruit salad for a balanced, nutritious meal. (Penny Lobdell, R.D.N., Kelowna, British Columbia)

Preparation: 15 minutes
Cook: 10 minutes
Makes 12 appetizer servings or 6 luncheon servings

Calories per pita: 312
Grams of protein per pita: 18.1
Grams of fat per pita: 13.2
Grams of carbohydrate per pita: 36.4
Grams of fibre per pita: 2.7

SALMON OASIS
Ellen Craig, Calgary, Alberta

Serve this filling on toasted English muffins: cut into quarters as an appetizer or serve whole for lunch.

4	whole wheat English muffins	4
1	can (7.5 oz./213 g) salmon	1
¼ cup	light mayonnaise	50 mL
2 tbsp.	finely chopped green onion	25 mL
2 tsp.	lemon juice	10 mL
½ tsp.	curry powder	2 mL
¼ tsp.	pepper	1 mL
8	green pepper strips	8
¾ cup	shredded low-fat mozzarella cheese	175 mL
	Paprika	

Split muffins in half and toast.

Combine salmon, mayonnaise, onion, lemon juice, curry powder, and pepper. Spread on muffin halves; top with green pepper and cheese. Sprinkle with paprika. Place on ungreased baking sheet. Broil about 3 minutes, or just until cheese melts.

MENU SUGGESTION
Teamed up with Manitoba Vegetable Soup (page 62), skim milk, and an apple, a Salmon Oasis lunch goes a long way towards meeting the daily requirement of almost every vitamin and mineral you can name, while keeping fat content down and fibre content high. (Elaine Power, R.Dt., Port aux Basques, Newfoundland)

Preparation: 10 minutes
Cook: about 3 minutes
Makes 8 servings

Calories per half muffin: 154
Grams of protein per half muffin: 10.6
Grams of fat per half muffin: 6.3
Grams of carbohydrate per half muffin: 13.3
Grams of fibre per half muffin: 1.8

LEMON PESTO SAUCE APPETIZERS
Margaret Howard, Toronto, Ontario

Here are three different appetizers made from the same basic pesto sauce. A good reason to make extra sauce and keep it on hand in the freezer.

PESTO PITA PIZZAS

½ cup	Lemon Pesto Sauce (page 177)	125 mL
2 tbsp.	grated Parmesan cheese	25 mL
3	whole wheat pita breads	3
½ cup	chopped red pepper	125 mL
1 cup	shredded low-fat mozzarella cheese	250 mL

Combine Lemon Pesto Sauce and Parmesan cheese. Cut each pita bread in half; then split each half (scissors make this step easier). Spread 1 tbsp. (15 mL) sauce over each split pita. Sprinkle with red pepper and mozzarella cheese. Bake in 450°F (230°C) oven for about 5 minutes, or until cheese melts.

Preparation: 15 minutes
Cook: 5 minutes
Makes 12 servings

Calories per serving: 97
Grams of protein per serving: 4.7
Grams of fat per serving: 4.5
Grams of carbohydrate per serving: 10.1
Grams of fibre per serving: 0.3

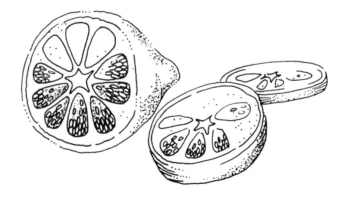

PESTO SPREAD

⅓ cup	light mayonnaise	75 mL
⅓ cup	finely chopped red pepper	75 mL
3 tbsp.	Lemon Pesto Sauce (page 177)	45 mL
3 tbsp.	grated Parmesan cheese	45 mL
1 ½ tsp.	Dijon mustard	7 mL
	Melba toast, pita bread, crackers Garnish: Lemon zest	

Makes about 1 cup (250 mL)
Serving size: 1 tbsp./15 mL

Calories per serving: 28
Grams of protein per serving: 0.6
Grams of fat per serving: 2.6
Grams of carbohydrate per serving: 0.9
Grams of fibre per serving: 0.1

In bowl, combine mayonnaise, red pepper, Lemon Pesto Sauce, cheese, and mustard. Serve spread on melba toast, pita wedges, or crackers. Garnish with fresh lemon zest.

PESTO DIP

¾ cup	low-fat plain yoghurt	175 mL
¼ cup	Lemon Pesto Sauce (page 177)	50 mL
	Melba toast, raw vegetables	

Preparation: 5 minutes
Makes 1 cup (250 mL)
Serving size: 1 tbsp./15 mL

Calories per serving: 17
Grams of protein per serving: 0.7
Grams of fat per serving: 1.1
Grams of carbohydrate per serving: 1.3
Grams of fibre per serving: 0

In bowl, combine yoghurt and Lemon Pesto Sauce. Serve with melba toast or raw vegetables.

Have you ever purchased an eggplant? It's easily recognized by its rich, purple-black colour. Eggplants have a very delicate skin, so treat them gently. Choose ones that are smooth and firm. Cook small eggplants whole. Stuff the larger ones or use them in casseroles. You can even substitute eggplant slices for noodles in your favourite lasagna recipe.

EGGPLANT TAPAS
Shirley Ann Holmes, Guelph, Ontario

In Spain, tapas are served as nibbles at bars, and as appetizers before dinner.

1	small eggplant (about ¾ lb./400 g)	1
1	medium green pepper	1
1	medium red pepper	1
2 tbsp.	lemon juice	25 mL
1 tbsp.	red wine vinegar	15 mL
1 tsp.	olive oil	5 mL
1	clove garlic, minced	1
	Freshly ground pepper	

Place eggplant and peppers on baking sheet. Bake in 400°F (200°C) oven for about 30 minutes, or until tender and peppers are charred. (Note: Peppers may be cooked before eggplant.) Allow to cool in a plastic bag. Placing peppers in plastic bag to cool will allow for easier handling and removal of skins. Remove skin from peppers and eggplant. Cut eggplant into chunks; cut peppers into thin slices.

Combine lemon juice, vinegar, oil, garlic, and pepper. Pour over vegetables and stir. Cover and refrigerate for several hours.

Preparation: 45 minutes
Chill: several hours
Makes 2 cups (500 mL) or 6 appetizer servings

Calories per serving: 104
Grams of protein per serving: 0.5
Grams of fat per serving: 0.9
Grams of carbohydrate per serving: 4.4
Grams of fibre per serving: 1.3

INGELEOGE VIS

Maddy Hoogstraten, Toronto, Ontario

This recipe stores beautifully—in fact, it is better made several days before serving. Keeps for up to 2 weeks in the refrigerator.

MARINADE

4	onions, sliced	4
¾ cup	raisins	175 mL
1½ cups	water	375 mL
½ cup	vinegar	125 mL
3 tbsp.	brown sugar	45 mL
1 tbsp.	dry mustard	15 mL
2 tsp.	curry powder	10 mL
½ tsp.	salt	2 mL
¼ tsp.	peppercorns	1 mL
2	bay leaves	2

2 lb.	fish fillets	1 kg
1 tsp.	curry powder	5 mL
1 tsp.	dried ginger	5 mL
1 tsp.	salt	5 mL
	Garnish: leaf lettuce, cherry tomatoes	

Cut fish into serving pieces. Sprinkle with curry powder, ginger, and salt. Bake in 425°F (220°C) oven for about 10 minutes, or until fish flakes easily with fork. Place fish in shallow bowl.

In small saucepan, combine onions, raisins, water, vinegar, brown sugar, and seasonings. Bring to boil; cook for 3 minutes. Pour over fish; cool slightly. Cover and refrigerate for 3 days; turn each day.

Serve as a starter on leaf lettuce with cherry tomatoes. Or for a more casual meal, serve in a dish surrounded by crackers and let guests help themselves.

MENU SUGGESTION

This dish, rich in protein while being low in fat, is delicious at the beginning of a meal. Follow it with Pasta with Broccoli Herb Sauce (page 172), Italian Broiled Tomatoes (page 122), and wild berries with yoghurt for a meal that offers a variety of taste, texture, and colour combinations. The broccoli and berries contribute fibre to the meal. (Darlene Witherall, R.Dt., St. John's, Newfoundland)

Preparation: 15 minutes
Cook: about 10 minutes
Makes 10 to 12 servings

Calories per serving: 108
Grams of protein per serving: 12.1
Grams of fat per serving: 0.9
Grams of carbohydrate per serving: 13.3
Grams of fibre per serving: 0.9

PIQUANT MARINATED VEGETABLES
The Canadian Dietetic Association

This intriguing combination of vegetables is best served as an appetizer salad on leaf lettuce, or as a side salad to a meat entrée. Make the entire recipe. It improves with time and keeps very well.

MARINADE

1 cup	red wine vinegar	250 mL
1 tsp.	dried oregano	5 mL
1 tsp.	dried tarragon	5 mL
½ tsp.	granulated sugar	2 mL
½ tsp.	salt	2 mL
¼ tsp.	freshly ground pepper	1 mL
¼ cup	olive oil	50 mL

2 cups	cauliflower florets	500 mL
2 cups	broccoli florets	500 mL
1 cup	fresh button mushrooms	250 mL
½	red pepper, cut into strips	½
1 cup	cut-up green beans	250 mL
8	small white pickling onions	8
1	carrot, cut into rounds	1

Lettuce leaves
Garnish: cherry tomatoes, chopped fresh parsley

In bowl, combine cauliflower, broccoli, mushrooms, red pepper, green beans, onions, and carrot.

To make marinade: In saucepan, heat vinegar and seasonings; add oil and pour over vegetables. Cool slightly and transfer mixture to a large plastic bag. Refrigerate for 24 hours before serving.

Serve in bowl lined with lettuce; garnish with cherry tomatoes and parsley. Provide toothpicks for spearing vegetables.

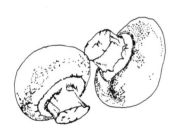

Preparation: about 20 minutes
Marinate: 24 hours or longer
Makes 10 servings

Calories per serving: 53
Grams of protein per serving: 2.0
Grams of fat per serving: 2.9
Grams of carbohydrate per serving: 6.5
Grams of fibre per serving: 2.8

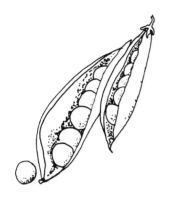

COTTAGE CHEESE HERB DIP
Marsha Sharp, Waterdown, Ontario

For best results, prepare this refreshing dip ahead of time and refrigerate overnight or longer. Serve with crudités (raw vegetables) to keep the calories low.

1 cup	low-fat (1 percent) cottage cheese	250 mL
½ cup	low-fat plain yoghurt	125 mL
1	green onion, chopped	1
½ tsp.	garlic powder	2 mL
½ tsp.	celery seed	2 mL
¼ tsp.	dry mustard	1 mL
¼ tsp.	Worcestershire sauce	1 mL
Pinch	pepper	Pinch
Dash	hot pepper sauce	Dash

Raw vegetables: broccoli, cauliflower, mushrooms, snow peas, green or red pepper, carrot, zucchini, or celery sticks.

In food processor or blender, cream cottage cheese and yoghurt until very smooth. Stir in onion and seasonings. Serve with raw vegetables.

MENU SUGGESTION

This low-fat, low-calorie dip will enhance any lazy afternoon picnic in the sun. A light spinach quiche adds to the protein for the meal and with the high-fibre accompaniment of raw vegetables, whole wheat rolls, and a fresh fruit salad, you have a well-balanced meal. (Jean Norman, R.Dt., St. John's, Newfoundland)

Preparation: 10 minutes
Chill: 24 hours
Makes 1½ cups (375 mL)
Serving size: 1 tbsp./15mL

Calories per serving: 11
Grams of protein per serving: 1.5
Grams of fat per serving: 0.2
Grams of carbohydrate per serving: 0.7
Grams of fibre per serving: 0

HOT VEGGIES AND GARLIC DIP

Denise Kilback, Balgonie, Saskatchewan

Tickle the eye and the appetite with this "prepare ahead but bake at serving time" starter. Serve hot vegetables for dunking in cold dip.

DIP

1 cup	low-fat plain yoghurt	250 mL
¼ cup	finely chopped green onion	50 mL
1	clove garlic, minced	1
1 tsp.	Dijon mustard	5 mL

¼ cup	buttermilk	50 mL
2 tbsp.	butter or margarine, melted	25 mL
2 tbsp.	Dijon mustard	25 mL
1 cup	whole wheat bread crumbs	250 mL
½ cup	grated Parmesan cheese	125 mL
Dash	freshly ground pepper	Dash
1	small eggplant, quartered	1
1	large zucchini	1
1	sweet onion	1

Combine buttermilk, butter, and mustard in shallow bowl.

Place bread crumbs, Parmesan cheese and pepper in plastic bag.

Cut vegetables ½ inch (1 cm) thick. Separate onion into rings. Dip vegetables into liquid, then shake in plastic bag to coat. Arrange vegetables on non-stick or lightly greased baking sheet. Bake in 400°F (200°C) oven for about 6 minutes; turn and bake for 5 minutes, or until golden brown.

To make dip: Combine yoghurt, onion, garlic, and mustard.

MENU SUGGESTION

A delicious and easy-to-prepare first course that's baked, not fried. The use of yoghurt rather than sour cream further minimizes the fat content. Follow it with poached salmon trout, brown rice pilaf, green beans with toasted almonds, tomato slices with vinegar and chopped basil, and Lemon Sherbet (page 224). (Barbara Burton, R.P.Dt., Gloucester, Ontario)

Preparation: 30 minutes
Cook: about 10 minutes
Makes 1 cup (250 mL) dip or 8 servings

Calories per serving: 149
Grams of protein per serving: 6.6
Grams of fat per serving: 5.7
Grams of carbohydrate per serving: 18.7
Grams of fibre per serving: 2.9

ORIENTAL CRAB SPREAD
Grissol

This delicious mixture, spread on melba toast, contains the flavours of the Far East and is a welcome addition to any before-dinner event.

⅓ cup	light cream cheese	75 mL
1 tbsp.	soy sauce	15 mL
1 tsp.	granulated sugar	5 mL
Dash	white pepper	Dash
1	can (120 g) crabmeat, drained	1
½ cup	finely chopped water chestnuts	125 mL
⅓ cup	finely chopped red pepper	75 mL
1	green onion, thinly sliced	1
2 tbsp.	low-fat plain yoghurt	25 mL
	Melba toast	

In small bowl, combine cream cheese, soy sauce, sugar, and pepper. Stir in crabmeat, water chestnuts, red pepper, onion, and yoghurt. Cover and refrigerate for 30 minutes or longer. Spread on melba toast.

Preparation: 10 minutes
Chill: 30 minutes or longer
Makes 1¾ cups (425 mL)
Serving size: 1 tbsp./15 mL

Calories per serving: 15
Grams of protein per serving: 1.2
Grams of fat per serving: 0.6
Grams of carbohydrate per serving: 1.1
Grams of fibre per serving: 0

SPINACH DIP
The Canadian Dietetic Association

A cool, clean-tasting, and, best of all, low-calorie dip that provides little fat because of its use of low-fat products. Enjoy it as a refreshing hors-d'oeuvre for relaxing moments. As a party dip, it will serve up to 20 guests.

Raw vegetables served with dips are popular at parties or as an appetizer. For an unusual conversation piece, use hollowed out peppers or half an acorn squash to hold your favourite dip recipe. Try some of the new, calorie-reduced, creamy salad dressings with your next vegetable tray, or mix yoghurt with herbs for an unusual dip.

1	package (300 g) frozen chopped spinach, thawed and drained	1
½ cup	chopped water chestnuts	125 mL
¼ cup	finely chopped onion	50 mL
¼ cup	chopped red pepper	50 mL
1	large clove garlic, mashed	1
1 cup	low-fat (1 percent) cottage cheese	250 mL
1 cup	low-fat plain yoghurt	250 mL
2 tsp.	dried basil	10 mL
¼ tsp.	dry mustard	1 mL
¼ tsp.	garlic powder	1 mL
	Freshly ground pepper	
	Round rye or pumpernickel bread	

In large bowl, combine spinach, water chestnuts, onion, red pepper and garlic. Stir in cottage cheese, yoghurt, and seasonings. Chill for several hours.

To serve, hollow out centre of bread. Cut bread into cubes; fill centre of bread with dip and surround with bread cubes.

Preparation: 15 minutes
Chill: at least 4 hours
Makes 4 cups (1 L) dip
Serving size: ¼ cup/50 mL

Calories per serving: 80
Grams of protein per serving: 4.6
Grams of fat per serving: 0.6
Grams of carbohydrate per serving: 14.9
Grams of fibre per serving: 1.1

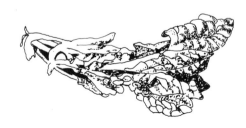

HUMMUS

Brenda Steinmetz, Toronto, Ontario

This less-oily version of the Middle Eastern dip uses yoghurt to replace much of the olive oil used in traditional hummus recipes. Serve as a dip with raw vegetable crudités or toasted pita-bread triangles.

1	can (19 oz./540 mL) chick peas, drained	1
2	green onions	2
2–4	large cloves garlic	2–4
¼ cup	fresh lemon juice	50 mL
¼ cup	tahini (sesame seed paste)*	50 mL
½ tsp.	ground cumin	2 mL
½ tsp.	salt	2 mL
	Freshly ground pepper	
½ cup	low-fat plain yoghurt	125 mL
	Garnish: chopped onion, tomato, and parsley	
	Raw vegetables, pita bread	

In food processor or blender, purée chick peas, green onions, garlic, lemon juice, tahini, and seasonings until smooth. Stir in yoghurt until well combined. Garnish with onion, tomato, and parsley.

Serve chilled or at room temperature with raw vegetables and pita bread.

Variation: Tofu Hummus sent in by Deborah Leach, St. John's, Newfoundland, replaces one-half of the chick peas with tofu and adds more tahini.

* Tahini is available in some super-markets and many health food and specialty stores. If you cannot find tahini, simply substitute toasted sesame seeds and process with chick peas.

PITA-HUMMUS SANDWICH

Stuff Hummus into split miniature or regular size pitas. You may wish to garnish this sandwich with a choice of raw vegetables like sliced radish, grated carrot, sliced cucumber, shredded lettuce, red cabbage, and alfalfa sprouts.

Preparation: 15 minutes
Chill: if desired
Makes 2¾ cups (675 mL)
Serving size: 1 tbsp./15 mL

Calories per serving: 55
Grams of protein per serving: 3.0
Grams of fat per serving: 1.3
Grams of carbohydrate per serving: 8.3
Grams of fibre per serving: 1.9

ORIENTAL PORK ROLLS WITH SWEET AND SOUR SAUCE

Rose Soneff, Penticton, British Columbia

Meatballs are always a popular appetizer, but when fried are high in fat. This version lets you use your microwave instead—healthier eating, and faster, too.

SAUCE

½ cup	crushed pineapple, drained	125 mL
½ cup	unsweetened pineapple juice	125 mL
⅓ cup	ketchup	75 mL
¼ cup	vinegar	50 mL
¼ cup	brown sugar	50 mL
4 tsp.	cornstarch	20 mL
2 tbsp.	water	25 mL

1 lb.	lean ground pork	500 g
1	can (4 oz./113 g) cocktail shrimp, drained	1
½ lb.	cooked ham, minced	250 g
½ cup	sliced water chestnuts, finely chopped	125 mL
½ cup	raisins, coarsely chopped	125 mL
4	green onions, chopped	4
2	garlic cloves, crushed	2
2	eggs, lightly beaten	2
2 tbsp.	all-purpose flour	25 mL
3 tbsp.	soy sauce	45 mL
2 tbsp.	chopped fresh coriander or	25 mL
1 tsp.	ground coriander	5 mL
	Garnish: fresh coriander	

These rolls freeze beautifully or may be refrigerated for up to three days ahead of the party. Sauces thickened with cornstarch are best made the day of the party as they could separate on reheating. Do not refrigerate the sauce, rather leave at room temperature, then reheat.

Combine pork, shrimp, ham, water chestnuts, raisins, onion, garlic, eggs, flour, soy sauce, and coriander. Roll into cylinders 6 inches (15 cm) long and 1 inch (2.5 cm) wide. Wrap in plastic wrap, then in waxed paper.

Microwave each roll on High (100 percent) for 4 to 5 minutes; rotate roll after 3 minutes. Allow to cool before cutting each roll into about 8 slices.

Preparation: 30 minutes
Cook: 5 minutes per roll
Makes 40 meat slices

Calories per meat slice with sauce: 60

Grams of protein per meat slice: 4.8

Grams of fat per meat slice: 2.1

Grams of carbohydrate per meat slice: 5.6

Grams of fibre per meat slice: 0.2

To make sauce: In saucepan, combine pineapple, juice, ketchup, vinegar, and brown sugar. Cook for about 5 minutes to dissolve sugar. Stir cornstarch into water; stir into hot mixture. Cook and stir for 3 minutes, or until thickened.

To serve, pour sauce onto serving dish; arrange meat slices on top. Garnish with sprigs of fresh coriander.

ARTICHOKE NUGGETS
Lena (Barrett) Putnam, Winsloe, P.E.I.

These freeze easily before baking and will be ready to serve at a moment's notice. To bake frozen, allow 5 minutes extra.

1	bottle (6 oz./170 mL) artichoke hearts, drained	1
½ cup	seasoned crouton crumbs (about 1 cup/250 mL croutons)	125 mL
1 tbsp.	olive oil	15 mL
1 tbsp.	grated Parmesan cheese	15 mL
1	egg, beaten	1
2 tsp.	lemon juice	10 mL
1	clove garlic, mashed	1
	Parmesan cheese	

Preparation: 15 minutes
Cook: 10 to 15 minutes
Makes 12 medium, 18 small nuggets

Calories per medium nugget: 45

Grams of protein per medium nugget: 2.0

Grams of fat per medium nugget: 2.4

Grams of carbohydrate per medium nugget: 3.9

Grams of fibre per medium nugget: 0.5

In small bowl, mash artichoke hearts. Stir in crouton crumbs, oil, cheese, egg, lemon juice, and garlic. Form into small balls. Roll each ball in additional Parmesan cheese (about ¼ cup/50 mL).

Bake in 350°F (180°C) oven for 10 minutes for small nuggets, 15 minutes for medium.

SOUPS

*Making soup from scratch
is easy, economical, and nutritious.
In fact, making soup stock is a superb
way to use unwanted meat trimmings
and raw vegetables past their prime,
as well as leftover bits and
pieces from meals.*

Soups are versatile. A hearty soup, like Beef Barley Soup (page 71) or Lakeshore Chowder (page 69) can be the base of a meal. A light soup, such as Iced Tomato Soup (page 64), provides a pleasant start to a traditional meal.

With homemade stock, soup certainly has more appetite appeal. Stock can also be used for sauces and entrées, for example, Lentil Spaghetti Sauce (page 107) or Fish Fillets with Basil Walnut Sauce (page 87).

Bones are the most important ingredient in any stock. They contribute flavour and substance. In recipes calling for chicken broth or stock, commercial products can also be substituted, but they generally are higher in sodium.

The Hodgepodge Pot method makes great soups. Keep a container in the refrigerator or freezer and consign any leftovers from the evening meal to the hodgepodge pot. When the pot is full, add some beef or chicken stock, simmer for a hearty soup without a name — or for that matter without a recipe. Each version will be a new experience.

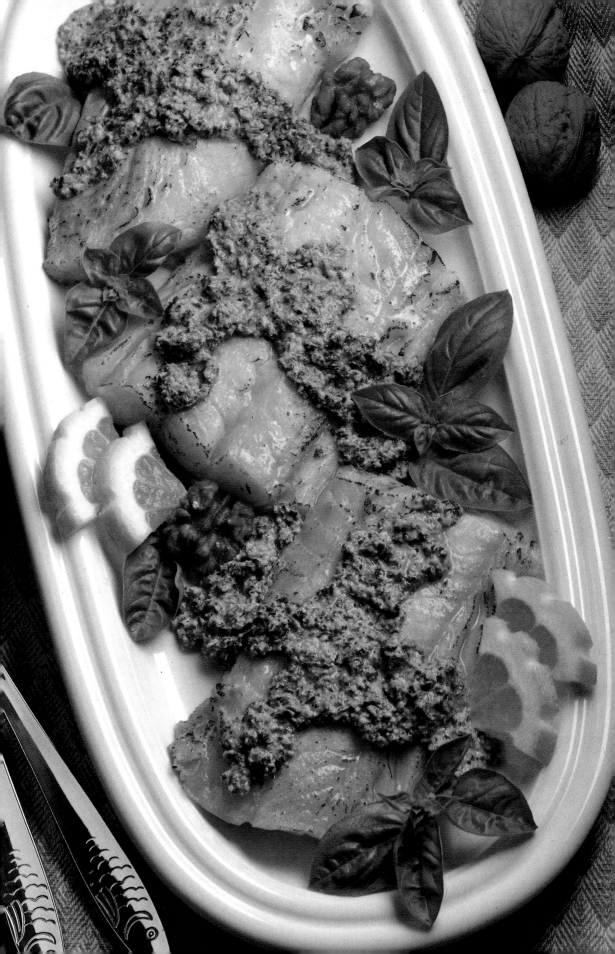

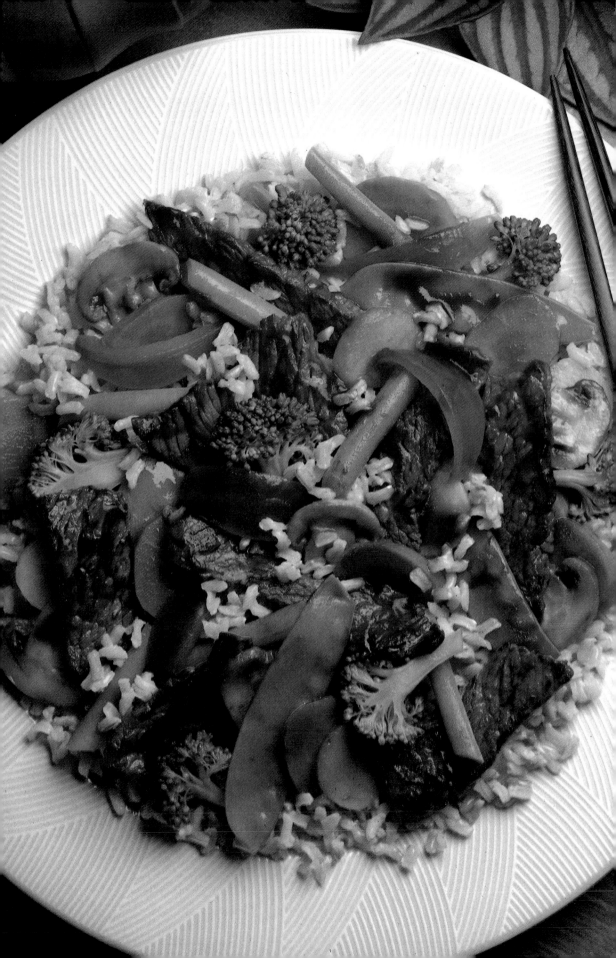

CHICKEN STOCK

3 lbs.	chicken*	1.5 kg
10 cups	water	2.5 L
3	sprigs parsley	3
1	onion, chopped	1
1	carrot, coarsely chopped (include peel)	1
1	stalk celery, coarsely chopped (include leaves)	1
1	leek, trimmed and cut up	1
1	bay leaf	1
½ tsp.	freshly ground pepper	2 mL
¼ tsp.	dried thyme	1 mL
¼ tsp.	dried marjoram	1 mL
	Salt to taste	

In large stockpot or Dutch oven, place chicken water, parsley, onion, carrot, celery, leek, and seasonings. Bring to boil; skim off foam. Cook covered, on low heat, for 1 to 3 hours, or until chicken is tender (depending on type of chicken used).

Remove chicken; reserve. Strain liquid through sieve; press down on vegetables to extract as much flavour as possible. Chill stock; remove fat from surface. Stock can be refrigerated for 2 to 3 days or frozen for up to 4 months. Reserved chicken can be used in different ways, depending on the type of meat used.

*You can use: 1. Chicken pieces (backs, necks, and wings): this is economical, and the small pieces of meat will provide flavour. The meat can be added to the hodgepodge pot after it is strained from stock. 2. Chicken parts: then you will have cooked chicken for another use (if you are saving the chicken for later use, cook it just until tender). 3. Stewing hen, for a wonderful flavour and some leftover chicken for other uses (this choice requires longest cooking time due to ''old age'' of the hen).

Preparation: 20 minutes   Cook: 1 to 3 hours
Makes 8 to 10 cups (2 to 2.5 L)

BEEF STOCK

3 lb.	meaty beef bones	1.5 kg
10 cups	water	2.5 L
3	sprigs parsley	3
2	onions, coarsely chopped	2
2	stalks celery, coarsely chopped (include leaves)	2
2	cloves garlic	2
1	carrot, coarsely chopped (include peel)	1
1	leek, trimmed and cut up	1
1	tomato, coarsely chopped	1
2	whole cloves	2
1	bay leaf	1
¼ tsp.	dried thyme	1 mL
¼ tsp.	peppercorns	1 mL
	Salt to taste	

In large shallow pan in 425°F (220°C) oven, roast bones for about 1 hour, or until well browned; turn occasionally. Transfer meat and bones to large stockpot or Dutch oven. Add water, parsley, onion, celery, garlic, carrot, leek, tomato, and seasonings. Bring to boil; skim off foam.

Cook covered, on low heat, for about 3 hours, or until meat is very tender. Lift out meat; reserve for another use. Remove bones and discard. Strain liquid through sieve; press down on vegetables to extract as much flavour as possible. Chill stock; remove fat from surface. Stock can be refrigerated for 2 to 3 days, or frozen for up to 4 months.

Preparation: 20 minutes
Cook: 4 hours
Makes about 8 cups (2 L)

Photos: Fish Fillets with Basil Walnut Sauce, page 87 (overleaf): Ginger Vegetable-Beef Medley, page 92 (facing page)

If Peter Piper picked a peck of pickled peppers today, he would be able to choose among red, green, yellow, and purple ones. We're most familiar with red and green peppers. A red pepper is a green one turned ripe. Large yellow peppers are also sweet and give an attractive colour to any dish. Sweet-flavoured purple peppers, common in Holland, are now being introduced in Canada.

MENU SUGGESTION

This versatile, quick-to-prepare soup has minimal fat and adds a touch of pizzazz to almost any menu, from a traditional roast beef dinner to a spicy Mexican meal. It provides lots of vitamin C. For a meal rich in fibre and low in fat, serve it followed by barbecued skinless lemon chicken (a good source of protein that keeps fat under control), with corn on the cob and roasted potatoes for additional fibre. Follow with kiwi sorbet. (Elaine Power, R.Dt., Port aux Basques, Newfoundland)

Preparation: 10 minutes
Chill: at least 3 hours
Makes 6 servings or 7 cups
(1.75 L)

Calories per serving: 52
Grams of protein per serving: 2.2
Grams of fat per serving: 0.4
Grams of carbohydrate per serving: 12.5
Grams of fibre per serving: 1.2

GAZPACHO
Deborah Leach, St. John's, Newfoundland

The Spaniards certainly know a good thing; they developed this wonderful cold soup for a hot climate. Our gazpacho is very low in fat and is easily prepared with a food processor or blender.

4 cups	tomato juice	1 L
⅓ cup	red wine vinegar	75 mL
1	medium green pepper, finely chopped	1
1	medium English cucumber, finely chopped	1
2	medium tomatoes, diced	2
1	small onion, chopped	1
2	cloves garlic, crushed	2
2 tbsp.	chopped chives	25 mL
¼ tsp.	paprika	1 mL

In large bowl, stir together tomato juice, vinegar, green pepper, cucumber, tomatoes, onion, garlic, chives, and paprika. Chill for 3 hours.

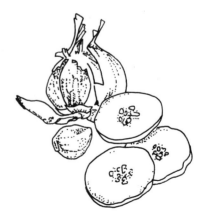

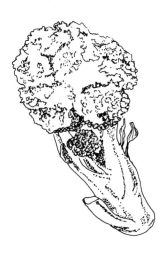

BABSI'S BROCCOLI SOUP
B.J. Rankin, Toronto, Ontario

This recipe was awarded honourable mention in the soup category of the CDA Healthy Eating Recipe Contest. It is a quick, yet unbelievably delicious and nutritious soup, which looks elegant when garnished. Make it all year round—serve it hot in winter and cold in summer.

2 cups	chopped broccoli, stems and florets	500 mL
2 cups	chicken broth	500 mL
1 cup	buttermilk	250 mL
½ tsp.	dried basil	2 mL
½ tsp.	dried tarragon	2 mL
	Salt and pepper to taste	
	Garnish: small broccoli florets, low-fat plain yoghurt, chives, shredded Cheddar cheese	

Cook broccoli in chicken broth for 10 minutes, or until tender. Refrigerate in broth until chilled.

In food processor or blender, purée chilled mixture, buttermilk, and seasonings until smooth. Taste to adjust seasonings. Reheat just to serving temperature, or chill and serve as cold soup. Serve garnished with broccoli, yoghurt, chives, and Cheddar cheese.

MENU SUGGESTION

Serve with Creamy Salmon Quiche (page 85), tossed green salad with low-fat dressing, whole wheat rolls, and fresh fruit for a meal that has almost half the recommended daily intake of calcium. Although the quiche has a higher fat content, it is balanced by these lower accompaniments. (Betty A. Brousse, R.P.Dt., Ottawa, Ontario)

Preparation: 10 minutes
Cook: 10 to 15 minutes
Chill: 2 hours
Makes 6 servings or about 3 cups (750 mL)

Calories per serving: 73
Grams of protein per serving: 6.7
Grams of fat per serving: 2.4
Grams of carbohydrate per serving: 7.3
Grams of fibre per serving: 1.9

SPICY PEANUT AND SPINACH SOUP
Selma Savage, Toronto, Ontario

Everyone who tries this unique and flavourful soup will ask for the recipe. Seasonings used are similar to those in Indian dishes. If this recipe is too large for your needs, freeze half before adding the spinach.

2	medium onions, chopped	2
2 tbsp.	chopped gingerroot	25 mL
1 cup	dry roasted, unsalted peanuts, chopped	250 mL
1	medium red pepper, chopped	1
1	medium green pepper, chopped	1
2	celery stalks, chopped	2
2	medium carrots, chopped	2
2	medium parsnips, chopped	2
1	small white turnip, chopped	1
2	small tomatoes, chopped	2
2	cloves garlic, minced	2
1 tsp.	ground cumin	5 mL
½ tsp.	ground coriander	2 mL
½ tsp.	turmeric	2 mL
½ tsp.	ground fennel	2 mL
¼ tsp.	ground cardamom	1 mL
2 tbsp.	vegetable oil	25 mL
4 cups	chicken broth	1 L
3 tbsp.	lemon juice	45 mL
2 tbsp.	brown sugar	25 mL
2 tsp.	soy sauce	10 mL
3 cups	packed, chopped spinach leaves	750 mL

MENU SUGGESTION

Don't let the name fool you—this soup tastes great and is full of nutrients. The vegetables are a rich source of vitamins and the peanuts add fibre and protein. Peanuts have a high fat content, so make sure the rest of the meal is low in fat. Serve with a whole wheat roll, Strawberry Sorbet (page 223), and milk for a nutritious lunch. (Janice Johnson, R.D.N., New Westminster, British Columbia)

Preparation: 20 minutes
Cook: 50 to 60 minutes
Makes 8 servings or 10 cups (2.5 L)

Calories per serving: 207

Grams of protein per serving: 8.8

Grams of fat per serving: 13.0

Grams of carbohydrate per serving: 16.9

Grams of fibre per serving: 4.0

In large stockpot on medium heat, cook onion, gingerroot, peanuts, peppers, celery, carrot, parsnip, turnip, tomato, garlic, and spices in hot oil for 10 minutes, or until softened. Add broth, lemon juice, sugar, and soy sauce; cook for about 35 minutes. Stir in spinach, cook for about 15 minutes.

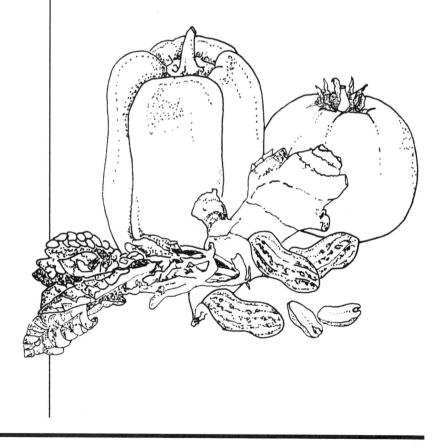

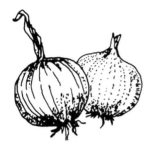

MANITOBA VEGETABLE SOUP
Lois Borkowsky, Teulon, Manitoba

Make this hearty soup when the days are cold and the larder is low.

4 cups	water	1 L
1	beef bouillon cube	1
1 cup	chopped potato	250 mL
1 cup	chopped carrot	250 mL
1 cup	chopped turnip	250 mL
⅓ cup	chopped celery	75 mL
⅓ cup	chopped onion	75 mL
1	can (14 oz./398 mL) tomatoes	1
1	can (14 oz./398 mL) kidney beans	1
½ tsp.	dried oregano	2 mL
½ tsp.	garlic powder	2 mL
½ tsp.	paprika	2 mL
	Salt and pepper to taste	
½ cup	cut-up green beans	125 mL

In large stockpot, combine water, bouillon cube, potato, carrot, turnip, celery, onion, tomatoes, kidney beans, and seasonings. Bring to a boil, reduce heat, cover and simmer for about 1 hour. Add green beans during last 10 minutes of cooking.

MENU SUGGESTION

This soup provides fibre with minimal fat. Complement it with chicken salad with almonds for protein. A whole wheat roll, lettuce and tomato salad, and fresh fruit for dessert provide extra fibre. (Roxanne Eyer, R.D., Winnipeg, Manitoba)

Preparation: 15 minutes
Cook: 1 hour
Makes 6 servings or approximately 7 cups (1.75 L)

Calories per serving: 114
Grams of protein per serving: 5.7
Grams of fat per serving: 0.6
Grams of carbohydrate per serving: 23.1
Grams of fibre per serving: 6.7

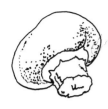

MUSHROOM, BROCCOLI, AND CORN CHOWDER

Victoria McKay, Woodstock, Ontario

A steaming bowl of chowder on a cold winter night provides a soothing start to a meal. Homemade chicken broth which has been defatted can be kept frozen for use in this recipe and others.

2 cups	chicken broth	500 mL
2	medium stalks broccoli, chopped	2
1 cup	sliced mushrooms	250 mL
½ cup	finely chopped onion	125 mL
2 tbsp.	butter or margarine	25 mL
2 tbsp.	all-purpose flour	25 mL
1½ cups	skim milk	375 mL
2 cups	whole kernel corn	500 mL
1 tbsp.	chopped pimento	15 mL

In large saucepan on medium heat, cook broth and broccoli for 5 minutes; set aside.

In skillet on medium-high heat, cook mushrooms and onion in butter for about 4 minutes, or until softened. Blend in flour; cook and stir for 2 minutes. Slowly add milk; cook and stir until smooth and thickened. Add broccoli mixture, corn, and pimento. Heat to serving temperature, or until corn and broccoli are cooked.

MENU SUGGESTION

This chowder contributes fibre, vitamins, and calcium. Serve it with a garden salad, Gib's Gourmet Muffins (page 192), and fresh fruit cup with Yorke Yoghurt (page 226) for additional protein and fibre. (Donna Law, R.D., Winnipeg, Manitoba)

To defat homemade chicken broth, refrigerate cooked broth until cold. Fat will solidify on surface and can be easily removed with a spoon or spatula.

Preparation: 10 minutes
Cook: 15 minutes
Makes 6 servings or 6 cups (1.5 L)

Calories per serving: 136
Grams of protein per serving: 7.2
Grams of fat per serving: 4.5
Grams of carbohydrate per serving: 19.4
Grams of fibre per serving: 3.4

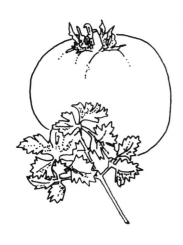

ICED TOMATO SOUP
Marion Elcombe, Edmonton, Alberta

On hot summer days, cold soups are very refreshing. On cold winter evenings, cold soups stimulate the appetite before a hot meal. For a richer version of this recipe, you can replace milk with cream. For a soup with less "bite," you can reduce the peppercorns.

1	can (19 oz./540 mL) tomatoes, divided	1
1¼ cups	2 percent milk	300 mL
1	can (10 oz./284 mL) condensed tomato soup	1
¼ cup	dry vermouth	50 mL
2 tbsp.	chopped green onion	25 mL
2 tbsp.	chopped red pepper	25 mL
2 tbsp.	chopped green pepper	25 mL
1 tbsp.	tomato paste	15 mL
1 tbsp.	peppercorns	15 mL
½ tsp.	dried oregano	2 mL
½ tsp.	Italian herb seasoning	2 mL
½ tsp.	granulated sugar	2 mL
	Garnish: Chopped green pepper, sliced green onions	

Preparation: 10 minutes
Chill: 3 hours
Makes 6 servings or 7 cups (1.75 L)

Calories per serving: 92
Grams of protein per serving: 3.3
Grams of fat per serving: 2.0
Grams of carbohydrate per serving: 14.2
Grams of fibre per serving: 0.8

In food processor or blender, combine half the tomatoes, milk, soup, vermouth, onion, peppers, and seasonings. Purée until smooth. Stir in reserved tomatoes; process for 3 to 5 seconds, so tomatoes remain chunky. Chill for about 3 hours.

Serve garnished with chopped green pepper and sliced green onions.

SPICY POTATO SOUP
F. Vautour, Moncton, New Brunswick

*For this unique potato soup, choose mild or hot green chilies
depending on the spice level you enjoy.*

2	large potatoes, cubed	2
2 cups	boiling water	500 mL
1	medium onion, finely chopped	1
1	medium green pepper, chopped	1
1	medium red pepper, chopped	1
2 tbsp.	butter or margarine	25 mL
¼ lb.	cooked ham, cubed	125 g
1 tbsp.	mild or hot green chilies	15 mL
¼ tsp.	white pepper	1 mL
1 cup	chicken broth	250 mL
1	egg yolk, slightly beaten	1
¼ cup	2 percent milk	50 mL
½ cup	shredded old Cheddar cheese (optional)	125 mL

In medium saucepan, cook potatoes in boiling water for
about 15 minutes, or until tender; drain and reserve liquid.

Sauté onion, green and red pepper in butter on medium
heat for 10 minutes, or until softened. Stir in ham, chilies,
and pepper; set aside.

In food processor or blender, purée cooked potatoes
with chicken broth until smooth. Return to saucepan with
reserved liquid; add vegetable mixture and reheat.

Beat egg yolk with milk, gradually stir into ½ cup (125
mL) hot soup. Return to saucepan. Heat gently, but do not
boil. Top with Cheddar cheese, if using.

MENU SUGGESTION
For a meal that's low in calories and rich in vitamins and minerals, serve this soup with Super Health Bread (page 189) and a citrus salad, which contributes fibre. Strawberry Yoghurt Pie (page 228) ends the meal with a delightful treat. (Jean Norman, R.Dt., St. John's, Newfoundland)

Preparation: 15 minutes
Cook: 25 to 30 minutes
Makes 6 servings or 7 cups (1.75 L)

Calories per serving: 147
Grams of protein per serving: 7.1
Grams of fat per serving: 6.6
Grams of carbohydrate per serving: 15.0
Grams of fibre per serving: 1.4

CURRIED SQUASH AND MUSHROOM SOUP

Anne M. Ferraro, Breadalbane, Prince Edward Island

Make this soup during the autumn when fresh squash is readily available. Or prepare year-round, using frozen mashed squash. Canned pumpkin or mashed cooked pumpkin can also be used.

MENU SUGGESTION

If you keep the first part of the meal low in fat, by serving this soup with red pepper salad and a whole wheat roll for fibre and skim-milk cheese for calcium and protein, you can splurge on Fruit Squares (page 198) for dessert with a clear conscience. (Jean Norman, R.Dt., St. John's, Newfoundland)

1	medium buttercup squash, peeled and chopped	1
½ lb.	sliced mushrooms	250 g
½ cup	chopped onions	125 mL
2 tbsp.	butter or margarine	25 mL
2 tbsp.	all-purpose flour	25 mL
1 tbsp.	curry powder	15 mL
5 cups	chicken broth	1.25 mL
½ cup	dry white wine or chicken broth	125 mL
1 tbsp.	honey	15 mL
Pinch	ground nutmeg	Pinch
1 cup	half-and-half (10 percent) cream, or 2 percent milk	250 mL

Preparation: 10 minutes
Cook: 20 minutes
Makes 6 servings or 7 cups (1.75 L)

Calories per serving with cream: 161
Grams of protein per serving: 6.6
Grams of fat per serving: 9.0
Grams of carbohydrate per serving: 14.6
Grams of fibre per serving: 1.8

Calories per serving with 2 percent milk: 135
Grams of protein per serving: 6.7
Grams of fat per serving: 5.9
Grams of carbohydrate per serving: 14.8
Grams of fibre per serving: 1.8

Steam squash until tender; purée in food processor until smooth.

In saucepan on medium-high heat, cook mushrooms and onions in butter until softened. Add flour and curry powder; cook and stir for 5 minutes. Gradually stir in chicken broth and wine; cook until smooth and slightly thickened. Whisk in squash, honey, and nutmeg; simmer for 15 minutes.

Stir in cream and reheat to serving temperature. Sprinkle with nutmeg and serve.

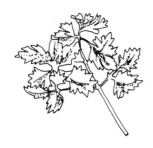

APPLE-WATERCRESS VICHYSSOISE
Goldie Moraff, Nepean, Ontario

Traditional vichyssoise is made with potatoes and leeks and served cold. This version adds Golden Delicious apples, apple juice, and fresh watercress. Try it hot for a change. All milk may be used for lower fat and fewer calories.

MENU SUGGESTION

Serve with roast pork, barley pilaf, Italian Broiled Tomatoes (page 122), and tossed green salad with low-fat dressing for a well-balanced meal. Enjoy fresh berries with low-fat yoghurt for dessert. (Tracy Darychuck, R.D.N., New Westminster, British Columbia)

2 cups	chicken broth	500 mL
1 cup	unsweetened apple juice	250 mL
2	large potatoes, chopped	2
2	large leeks, sliced (white part only)	2
2	Golden Delicious apples, peeled and chopped	2
¼ tsp.	ground cumin	1 mL
½ cup	packed fresh watercress leaves	125 mL
1 cup	2 percent milk	250 mL
1 cup	light cream or milk	250 mL
	Salt and white pepper to taste	
	Garnish: watercress sprigs, diced red apple	

Preparation: 15 minutes
Cook: about 25 minutes
Chill: 2 hours
Makes 8 servings or approximately 6 cups (1.5 L)

Calories per serving using half milk and half cream: 139
Grams of protein per serving: 4.2
Grams of fat per serving: 4.1
Grams of carbohydrate per serving: 22.4
Grams of fibre per serving: 1.9

Calories per serving using all 2 percent milk: 119
Grams of protein per serving: 4.3
Grams of fat per serving: 1.7
Grams of carbohydrate per serving: 22.5
Grams of fibre per serving: 1.9

In covered saucepan on medium heat, cook chicken broth, apple juice, potatoes, leeks, apples, and cumin for about 25 minutes, or until all ingredients are soft. Remove from heat; cool slightly.

In blender or food processor, purée potato mixture until smooth. Add watercress leaves and process just until chopped (do not overprocess). Add milk, cream, salt, and pepper; mix well. Chill for about 2 hours. Serve garnished with sprigs of watercress and a few apple pieces.

FISH AND VEGETABLE MEDLEY
Elaine Watton, Corner Brook, Newfoundland

This Maritime recipe features cod, which is readily available in Newfoundland. You can substitute other solid whitefish, like turbot, halibut, or haddock.

1	large onion, chopped	1
1	clove garlic, minced	1
2 tbsp.	butter or margarine	25 mL
1 cup	green pepper strips (or green and red pepper mixed)	250 mL
1 cup	cauliflower florets	250 mL
1 cup	broccoli florets	250 mL
1 cup	chopped tomato	250 mL
½ cup	chopped celery	125 mL
1 tbsp.	chopped fresh parsley	15 mL
1 lb.	cod fillets, cut into chunks	500 g
2½ cups	hot chicken broth	625 mL
1 tsp.	salt	5 mL
¼ tsp.	dried thyme	1 mL
¼ tsp.	dried basil	1 mL
¼ tsp.	freshly ground black pepper	1 mL

In large saucepan on medium heat, cook onion and garlic in butter for 3 minutes. Add pepper strips, cauliflower, broccoli, tomato, celery, and parsley; cook for 2 minutes. Add fish; cover, and cook for 2 minutes. Add chicken broth and seasonings and simmer for about 5 minutes, or until fish flakes with a fork and vegetables are crisp-tender.

MENU SUGGESTION

This soup is rich in protein, fibre, and vitamins. For a hearty meal, serve it with cucumber vinaigrette and homemade whole wheat bread. Buttermilk Oat-Branana Cake (page 235) for dessert will satisfy even the largest appetite. (Jeanine Chiasson, R.Dt., St. John's, Newfoundland)

Preparation: 15 minutes
Cook: about 10 minutes
Makes 4 to 6 servings or about 6 cups (1.5 L)

Calories per serving: 191
Grams of protein per serving: 22.8
Grams of fat per serving: 8.0
Grams of carbohydrate per serving: 6.6
Grams of fibre per serving: 2.1

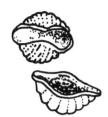

LAKESHORE CHOWDER
Kay Miskiw, Vegreville, Alberta

This easy and nutritious recipe will come in handy for a last-minute supper since it uses foods on hand in your cupboard.

½ cup	small pasta shells	125 mL
3 cups	boiling water	750 mL
1	large potato, diced	1
1	bay leaf	1
½ tsp.	salt	2 mL
¼ tsp.	coarsely ground pepper	1 mL
1	large onion, finely chopped	1
1	stalk celery, finely chopped	1
2 tbsp.	butter or margarine	25 mL
2 tbsp.	all-purpose flour	25 mL
3 cups	2 percent milk	750 mL
1	can (5 oz./142 mL) baby clams, drained	1
1	can (6.5 oz./184 g) flaked tuna, packed in water, drained	1
½ cup	whole kernel corn	125 mL
½ tsp.	curry powder	2 mL

MENU SUGGESTION

For a heart-warming supper on a cold winter night, serve this nutritious chowder with multi-grain or rye buns with cheese spread and raw vegetable crudités. The cheese spread provides protein and calcium with minimal fat. Finish the meal with Yorke Yoghurt (page 226). (Penny Lobdell, R.D.N., Kelowna, British Columbia)

Preparation: 15 minutes
Cook: 20 to 25 minutes
Makes 8 servings or 8 cups (2 L)

Calories per serving: 165
Grams of protein per serving: 11.9
Grams of fat per serving: 4.9
Grams of carbohydrate per serving: 18.3
Grams of fibre per serving: 1.1

In large pot, cook pasta in water for 5 minutes. Add potato, bay leaf, salt, and pepper; simmer for about 10 minutes, or until potatoes are tender.

In skillet on high heat, cook onion and celery in butter. Add flour; cook and stir for about 3 minutes. Stir in milk. Cook until thickened and sauce is smooth. Add to potato mixture. Add clams, tuna, corn, and curry powder to soup. Reheat to serving temperature; remove bay leaf.

HAMBURGER SOUP
Paula Worton, Espanola, Ontario

This hearty family-style soup makes a complete meal when pasta or barley are added. For a first course or luncheon soup, omit the pasta. The recipe makes a large quantity, but it freezes well.

1 lb.	lean ground beef	500 g
1	can (28 oz./798 mL) tomatoes	1
1	can (19 oz./540 mL) kidney beans	1
1	can (10 oz./284 mL) condensed tomato soup	1
5 cups	water	1.25 L
1	medium onion, chopped	1
1	carrot, chopped	1
½ cup	chopped celery	125 mL
½ cup	sliced mushrooms	125 mL
1 tsp.	Worcestershire sauce	5 mL
¼ tsp.	hot pepper sauce	1 mL
¼ tsp.	freshly ground pepper	1 mL
2	small zucchini, chopped	2

In large stockpot on medium heat, brown beef until crumbly; drain fat. Add tomatoes, kidney beans, tomato soup, water, onion, carrot, celery, mushrooms, and seasonings. Bring to boil. Reduce heat, and simmer covered for about 35 minutes. Add zucchini. Simmer 10 minutes longer.

Variations: Uncooked pasta or barley—about ½ cup (125 mL)—may be added for a more robust meal. For barley, add with vegetables and cook for 35 minutes. For pasta, add with zucchini and cook for 10 minutes.

MENU SUGGESTION

Complement this robust mix of vegetables, beef, pasta, and beans rich in vitamins and fibre with whole wheat mini loaves and vegetable crudités. An assorted cheese tray contributes sufficient protein to the meal. Round out the meal with peach bread pudding. (Yolanda Jakus, R.P.Dt., London, Ontario)

Preparation: 15 minutes
Cook: about 45 minutes
Makes 12 servings or 12 cups (3 L)

Calories per serving: 145
Grams of protein per serving: 10.9
Grams of fat per serving: 4.8
Grams of carbohydrate per serving: 15.3
Grams of fibre per serving: 4.2

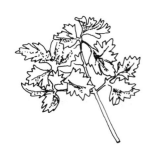

BEEF BARLEY SOUP
Karen Dewar, Teulon, Manitoba

Karen Dewar also sent us a recipe for hearty Whole Wheat Biscuits (page 190) to be served with this satisfying soup.

3½ cups	water	875 mL
¾ cup	tomato sauce	175 mL
¾ cup	dried soup mix (lentils, split peas, barley)	175 mL
1	beef bouillon cube	1
1	medium carrot, diced	1
1	medium potato, diced	1
2 tsp.	dried basil	10 mL
½ tsp.	salt	2 mL
¼ tsp.	freshly ground pepper	1 mL
½ cup	cubed cooked lean beef	125 mL

In large stockpot, combine water, tomato sauce, dried soup mix, bouillon cube, carrot, potato, and seasonings. Bring to boil. Reduce heat and simmer, covered, for about 1 hour. Add beef. Cook 30 minutes longer.

MENU SUGGESTION

This soup contributes protein and fibre with minimal fat, and is a good source of iron. Serve with warm Whole Wheat Biscuits (page 190), crunchy and colourful raw vegetables, an apple, and 2 percent milk for a nutritious meal that meets Canada's Food Guide. (Penny Lobdell, R.D.N., Kelowna, British Columbia)

Dried soup mix is available in bulk or health-food stores as well as in the supermarket.

Preparation: 15 minutes
Cook: 1 to 1½ hours
Makes 4 servings or 4 cups (1 L)

Calories per serving: 194
Grams of protein per serving: 12.7
Grams of fat per serving: 1.9
Grams of carbohydrate per serving: 32.8
Grams of fibre per serving: 5.3

MAIN COURSES

You will find an interesting array of main courses in this section—Oriental, Italian, and Indian dishes; fish, pork, poultry, lamb, and beef—something to suit everyone's taste.

Fragrant herbs and spices accent the natural flavours of meats, allowing you to cook using one of the lower-fat methods —grilling, stir-frying, broiling, roasting, or braising. These methods also help retain natural juices and flavour. Another way to enhance the flavour of meat is to use a marinade. In some cases, these will also tenderize meats. See marinades (page 97).

Let's look at each kind of meat separately.

POULTRY

Poultry takes on a different character depending on the company it keeps. This versatile and relatively inexpensive meat is a favourite of busy cooks. Remember to remove the skin before cooking to cut the fat content. Also remember that white meat is leaner than dark.

Ground chicken and turkey, now becoming available in supermarkets across the country, can add variety to meat loaves, patties, meatballs, quick stir-fries, like Turkiaki Fiesta (page 83), and more traditional recipes, like Chicken-Vegetable Lasagna (page 78).

How To Select Poultry: Choose fresh or frozen poultry that is tightly wrapped and is free of tears. When buying raw poultry, remember that 1 lb. (500 g) provides 3 to 4 servings.

How To Store Poultry: Fresh poultry: remove giblets and refrigerate them; use giblets within 2 days. Store poultry, loosely covered, in the coldest part of refrigerator; cook poultry within 3 days. Stuff poultry just before cooking.

Frozen poultry: keep frozen in original wrapper until time to thaw it for cooking. Frozen whole poultry can be kept for up to one year; poultry parts for up to 6 months. After thawing, do not refreeze until cooked.

Cooked poultry: store cooked poultry in the coldest part of refrigerator for up to 4 days or in freezer for up to 1 month. Remove stuffing from poultry immediately after cooking; store stuffing, refrigerated, in a separate container.

How To Thaw Frozen Poultry: Refrigerator: thaw poultry in the refrigerator; allow 5 hours per pound (10 hours per kilogram).
Cold water: cover poultry with cold water. Change water occasionally. Allow 1 hour per pound (2 hours per kilogram).
Microwave: follow directions in manufacturer's manual. Thaw on defrost setting.

Cook poultry immediately after thawing.

SEAFOOD AND FISH

Seafood, with its quick and easy preparation, is enjoying an even brighter spotlight these days. Proper cooking techniques ensure that the fish remains moist, tender, and flaky. Do not overcook, however. Seafood can be cooked using a variety of methods. From grilling, barbecuing, and broiling to microwaving and poaching, the recipes in this section are perfect choices for light, and easy cooking. Use high heat and a short cooking time.

The Canadian Department of Fisheries has developed a guide for fish cookery: measure fish at its thickest point and bake 10 minutes per inch (2.5 cm) of thickness in 450°F (230°C) oven. Double cooking time if fish is frozen. The same rule applies for poaching, broiling, and grilling. When done, fish will be opaque and will flake easily.

In the microwave, cook 1 pound (500 g) of thawed fish on High (100 percent) for 4 to 5 minutes. Always allow to stand for at least 5 minutes. For further directions, consult a microwave cookbook.

Some fish are best suited to baking and broiling; some are perfect for poaching. A general rule of thumb: thin fish should be broiled, grilled, microwaved, or barbecued. Thick fish, like whole fish or thick fillets, are better when baked or poached.

How To Select Fish: When buying fish, be sure to check for freshness. To do this, check the following:
- The eyes must be bright, clear, and bulging.
- Gills should be reddish or pink and fresh smelling.
- Scales should be shiny and tight to the skin.
- Fish should be firm and spring back when pressed.
- There should never be a strong or unpleasant odour.

To judge the amount to buy, remember, you will need ¼ lb. (125 g) of edible fish per person. To get this, you generally must buy ½ lb. (250 g) of unfilleted fish.

BEEF, PORK, AND LAMB
Tender cuts of beef from the loin, sirloin, and rib areas usually contain more fat and are higher in calories than those from the round, chuck, and flank. Buy leaner, less tender cuts with less marbling, and always trim all visible fat before cooking.

Marinating less tender cuts in an acid, such as vinegar, lemon juice, wine, or beer will increase the flavour and tenderness. (See marinades page 97.)

Herb and Spice Storage Tips

Here are several easy rules to follow:
- Store herbs and spices in tightly sealed containers in a dark location, away from heat, light, and moisture.
- Do not pour herbs or spices directly from the container into a steaming pot, as moisture will get trapped inside the container.
- Close the container as soon as you've finished using it.
- Be sure to replace herbs on a regular basis. Their optimum shelf life, after opening, is one year.
- Taste before, during, and after cooking.
- Bulk spices may not always the best buy. They are sometimes stale from having been stored in a large open bin.

CHICKEN PIZZA
Marlyn Ambrose-Chase, Moose Jaw, Saskatchewan

Pizza, everyone's perennial favourite, gets a new look in this recipe. Keep pizza dough rounds in the freezer to make this recipe quickly or make your own homemade dough or Whole Wheat Pizza Dough (page 187).

(page 187).

MENU SUGGESTION

Since this pizza, which is rich in protein, calcium, and B vitamins, has almost 40 percent of its calories from fat, serve it with foods that are low in fat. Raw vegetable sticks and lemon sherbet round out the meal. (Joanne Franko, P.Dt., Saskatoon, Saskatchewan)

1	12-inch (30 cm) pizza dough round, prepared or homemade	1
⅓ cup	tomato paste	75 mL
⅓ cup	water	75 mL
1 tbsp.	vegetable oil	15 mL
½ tsp.	dried oregano	2 mL
¼ tsp.	celery seed	1 mL
Dash	hot pepper sauce	Dash
Pinch	black pepper	Pinch
1 cup	sliced mushrooms	250 mL
1 cup	diced cooked chicken	250 mL
½ cup	diced canned pineapple	125 mL
¼ cup	minced ham (optional)	50 mL
¼ cup	diced green pepper	50 mL
1½ cups	shredded low-fat mozzarella cheese	375 mL
2 tbsp.	grated Parmesan cheese	25 mL
	Oregano and celery seed	

Preparation: 15 minutes
Cook: 12 to 15 minutes
Makes 6 servings

Calories per serving: 245
Grams of protein per serving: 17.0
Grams of fat per serving: 10.4
Grams of carbohydrate per serving: 21.1
Grams of fibre per serving: 1.9

Place pizza dough round on large baking sheet. Combine tomato paste, water, oil, and seasonings. Spread over dough. Arrange mushrooms, chicken, pineapple, ham (if using), and green pepper on top. Top with mozzarella and Parmesan cheese. Sprinkle with oregano and celery seed. Bake in 350°F (180°C) oven for 12 to 15 minutes. Cut into wedges to serve.

CREAMY MUSTARD CHICKEN
Diane Felker, Victoria, British Columbia

The combination of Dijon mustard and yoghurt in this recipe creates a light sauce with a French flair. Serve it with cooked white or wild rice.

MENU SUGGESTION

The rich, tangy sauce makes this recipe higher in fat. Balance out the meal with lower-fat foods, such as brown or wild rice, Deluxe Peas (page 125), steamed carrots, and fresh fruit salad, which contribute complex carbohydrates and fibre. (Tina L. Hartnell, R.D.N., Burnaby, British Columbia)

2 lb.	chicken pieces, skinned	1 kg
½ cup	low-fat plain yoghurt	125 mL
⅓ cup	light mayonnaise	75 mL
¼ cup	sliced green onions	50 mL
1 tbsp.	Dijon mustard	15 mL
1 tbsp.	Worcestershire sauce	15 mL
½ tsp.	dried thyme	2 mL
½ tsp.	salt	2 mL
¼ tsp.	white pepper	1 mL
2 tbsp.	grated Parmesan cheese	25 mL
	Garnish: chopped fresh parsley	

Place chicken in single layer in lightly greased, oven-proof casserole. Combine yoghurt, mayonnaise, onions, mustard, and seasonings. Spoon sauce over each chicken piece. Bake in 350°F (180°C) oven for about 45 minutes, or until chicken is tender. Sprinkle with Parmesan cheese and brown under the broiler. Serve garnished with chopped parsley.

Preparation: 10 minutes
Cook: 45 minutes
Makes 5 to 6 servings

Calories per serving: 217
Grams of protein per serving: 25.0
Grams of fat per serving: 11.1
Grams of carbohydrate per serving: 3.2
Grams of fibre per serving: 0.1

CHICKEN AND BROCCOLI BAKE
Patrick Mullin, Sault Ste. Marie, Ontario

Most good cooks agree that making a casserole the day before improves the flavours. Sautéing the chicken first speeds up the cooking, and overcooking toughens the meat.

MENU SUGGESTION

This one-dish meal combines foods from all four groups of Canada's Food Guide. A tossed green salad with herb vinaigrette dressing and a light peach and berry crisp for dessert adds colour and fibre. (Rooksana R. Willemsen, R.P.Dt., Fort Frances, Ontario)

6	chicken breast halves, skinned and boned	6
1	green onion, finely chopped	1
3 tbsp.	butter or margarine	45 mL
2 tsp.	lemon juice	10 mL
3 tbsp.	all-purpose flour	45 mL
2 cups	2 percent milk	500 mL
1 tbsp.	chopped fresh parsley	15 mL
½ tsp.	salt	2 mL
¼ tsp.	dried basil	1 mL
Pinch	pepper	Pinch
1 cup	shredded Cheddar cheese, divided	250 mL
1 cup	egg noodles	250 mL
2	medium tomatoes, sliced	2
2 cups	chopped broccoli, blanched	500 mL

Prevent Food Poisoning
To help reduce the risk of food poisoning in your kitchen:
- wash your hands before and after handling food, especially raw meat, fish, or poultry
- use a polyethylene cutting board for raw meat, fish, and poultry
- keep hot food hot (140°F/ 60°C) and cold food cold (40°F/4°C)
- never serve undercooked poultry

In large skillet on medium-high heat, cook chicken and onion in butter on one side until golden brown. Turn chicken to brown other side; sprinkle with lemon juice. Remove chicken. Whisk flour into pan juices; cook and stir for 2 minutes. Gradually whisk in milk, stirring constantly until smooth and thickened. Stir in seasonings and half the cheese.

In large pot of boiling water, cook noodles according to package directions, or until *al dente* (tender but firm); drain well. Place cooked noodles in a lightly greased,

Preparation: 15 minutes
Cook: 30 to 35 minutes
Makes 6 servings

Calories per serving: 384
Grams of protein per serving:
37.8
Grams of fat per serving: 17.1
Grams of carbohydrate per
serving: 19.6
Grams of fibre per serving: 2.2

oblong baking dish. Top with half the sauce. Arrange
tomato slices, broccoli, and chicken on top of noodles.
Cover with remaining sauce. Sprinkle with remaining
cheese. Bake, uncovered, in 350°F (180°C) oven for
about 30 minutes.

Variation: Daniel Déry, Ottawa, Ontario sent in a similar
recipe and suggested the Cheddar cheese could be
replaced with Swiss cheese.

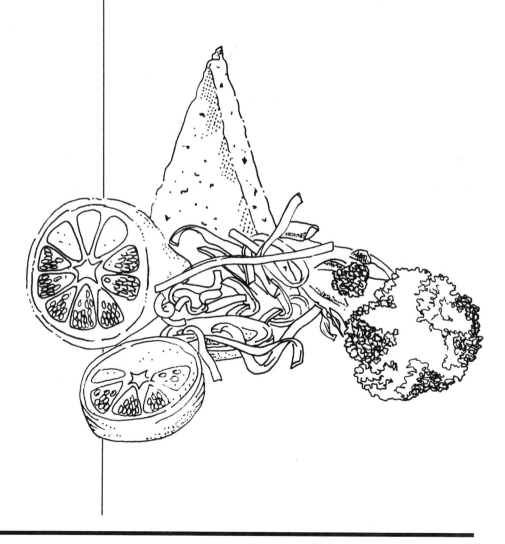

CHICKEN-VEGETABLE LASAGNA

Lisa Raitano, Etobicoke, Ontario

Lasagna is the hands-down favourite pasta dish for parties. This chicken and vegetable lasagna is light but satisfying and less expensive than more traditional lasagnas.

MENU SUGGESTION

This is a lower-fat, higher-fibre alternative to traditional lasagna. Chicken provides the protein. Replacing the usual eggs and cottage cheese with vegetables lowers the fat and adds extra fibre and vitamins. Serve it with spinach salad, Grandma's Unsweetened Rolled Oat Cookies (page 194), and skim milk. (Janice Johnson, R.D.N., New Westminster, British Columbia)

½ lb.	lean ground chicken	250 g
½ cup	chopped onion	125 mL
2	cloves garlic, minced	2
1 tbsp.	vegetable oil	15 mL
1 tsp.	butter or margarine	5 mL
1	can (28 oz./796 mL) tomatoes	1
1	can (5 ½ oz./156 mL) tomato paste	1
¾ cup	water	175 mL
1 ½ tsp.	salt	7 mL
Pinch	black pepper	Pinch
4	medium carrots, diced	4
1	bunch broccoli, chopped	1
½ lb.	mushrooms, sliced	250 g
¼ cup	chopped fresh parsley	50 mL
¾ lb.	lasagna noodles	375 g
1	package (6 oz./180 g) sliced low-fat mozzarella cheese	1
	Parmesan cheese	

In saucepan, on medium-high heat, cook chicken, onion, and garlic in oil and butter until all pink colour in chicken has disappeared. Add tomatoes, tomato paste, water, salt, and pepper. Cook, uncovered, on medium heat for about 15 minutes; stir occasionally.

Preparation: 20 minutes
Cook: about 30 minutes
Makes 8 servings

Calories per serving: 348
Grams of protein per serving: 20.9
Grams of fat per serving: 8.6
Grams of carbohydrate per serving: 48.5
Grams of fibre per serving: 5.5

Add carrots, broccoli, mushrooms, and parsley. Cook, covered, on low heat for about 30 minutes, or until mixture is thickened.

In large pot of boiling water, cook lasagna according to package directions, or until *al dente* (tender yet firm); drain well.

Spoon one-quarter of the sauce into 9 × 13-inch (3.5 L) baking dish. Place one-third of lasagna noodles over sauce. Repeat layers twice, ending with sauce. Top with cheese slices; sprinkle lightly with Parmesan cheese. Bake in 350°F (180°C) oven for about 30 minutes. Let stand 10 minutes before serving.

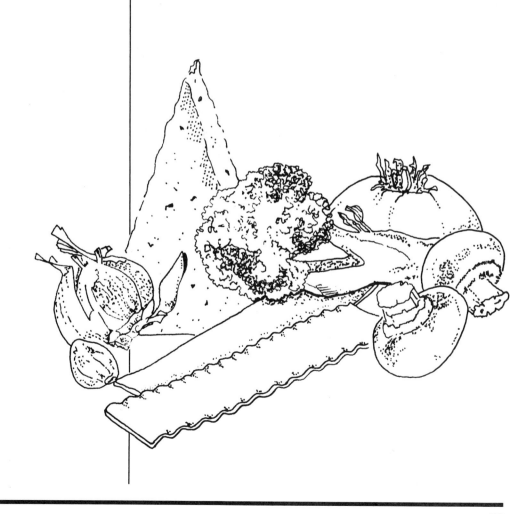

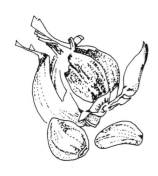

TANGY GLAZED CHICKEN
Kay Dallimore, Weston, Ontario

Apricot jam or orange marmalade, combined with flavours of the Far East, lends an imported flair to this chicken dish.

1 lb.	chicken breasts, skinned and boned	500 g
2 tbsp.	sugar-reduced apricot jam or orange marmalade	25 mL
2 tbsp.	unsweetened orange juice	25 mL
1	small clove garlic, minced	1
2 tsp.	soy sauce	10 mL
½ tsp.	ground ginger	2 mL
¼ tsp.	dry mustard	1 mL

Place chicken in shallow, non-stick or lightly greased baking pan. Combine jam, orange juice, garlic, soy sauce, and seasonings. Spoon sauce over chicken. Bake in 350°F (180°C) oven for about 45 minutes, or until chicken is tender and lightly glazed.

MENU SUGGESTION

This is a good dish for the weight-conscious eater. To keep the meal low in fat and calories, serve with fibre-rich brown rice, steamed green beans, marinated tomatoes, and finish with lime sherbet topped with fresh berries. (Marion Musial, R.D., Calgary, Alberta)

Preparation: 5 minutes
Cook: about 45 minutes
Makes 4 servings

Calories per serving: 151
Grams of protein per serving: 26.1
Grams of fat per serving: 3.0
Grams of carbohydrate per serving: 3.0
Grams of fibre per serving: 0

TURKEY HAZELNUT ROLL
Denise Giguere, Montreal, Quebec

To obtain firm slices of this nutty roll, cook the night before and refrigerate. The next day, slice the chilled roll and reheat slices in oven, or microwave at low heat, making sure they are well covered.

½	turkey breast, boned and halved lengthwise	½
1	turkey thigh, boned	1
½ cup	whole hazelnuts	125 mL
½ cup	wheat germ	125 mL
1 tbsp.	brandy or cognac	15 mL
1	egg, beaten	1
1 tsp.	salt	5 mL
1 tsp.	dried thyme	5 mL
½ tsp.	pepper	2 mL
	Cranberry sauce	

Flatten boned turkey breast pieces by pounding between two sheets of heavy plastic wrap. Cut one-third of turkey thigh into ½-inch (1 cm) cubes. Grind remaining two-thirds of turkey thigh to the consistency of minced meat.

In bowl, combine ground turkey with turkey cubes, hazelnuts, wheat germ, brandy, egg, and seasonings. Spread mixture over one flattened turkey breast and cover with the other to form a sandwich. Sew the edges of the sandwich closed with needle and thread. Roll up; tie with string like a roast; wrap in aluminum foil (dull side on the outside) to form an airtight seal.

Place turkey roll in baking pan containing 1 inch (2.5 cm) boiling water. Bake, uncovered, in 350°F (180°C) oven for 1½ hours. Slice and serve with cranberry sauce.

MENU SUGGESTION
This nutty roll is perfect for festive occasions. Complement it with baked potatoes, steamed baby Brussels sprouts, Hawaiian Cranberry Salad (page 140), and whole wheat rolls for added fibre. Serve Pumpkin Custard (page 214) for dessert. (Laurel Temple, R.D., Medicine Hat, Alberta)

Preparation: 30 minutes
Cook: 1½ hours
Makes 4 to 6 servings

Calories per serving: 208
Grams of protein per serving: 22.6
Grams of fat per serving: 9.7
Grams of carbohydrate per serving: 7.1
Grams of fibre per serving: 2.0

TURKEY CUTLETS WITH SUNSHINE SAUCE

Linda Terra, Calgary, Alberta

A delicious blend of flavours makes this nutritious and colourful dish unique. Calories and fat are kept in check by using orange juice and vegetables in the sauce and by using minimal oil for frying.

SUNSHINE SAUCE

2	green onions, finely chopped	2
2 tbsp.	butter or margarine	25 mL
2 cups	water	500 mL
2 tbsp.	cornstarch	25 mL
¼ cup	frozen concentrated orange juice, thawed	50 mL
2	chicken bouillon cubes, crumbled	2
1 cup	finely grated carrot	250 mL
1 tsp.	grated orange peel	5 mL
	Salt and pepper to taste	

6	turkey or chicken cutlets	6
1 cup	buttermilk	250 mL
2 cups	fine dry bread crumbs	500 mL
2 tbsp.	grated Parmesan cheese	25 mL
1 tsp.	paprika	5 mL
½ tsp.	salt	2 mL
¼ tsp.	garlic powder	1 mL
¼ tsp.	dried thyme	1 mL
¼ tsp.	ground turmeric	1 mL
¼ tsp.	dried rosemary	1 mL
¼ tsp.	pepper	1 mL
2 tbsp.	vegetable oil	25 mL

Dip turkey pieces into buttermilk. Combine bread crumbs, cheese, and seasonings. Dip turkey into bread-crumb mixture, coating thoroughly on all sides.

In large skillet on medium-high heat, brown turkey in hot oil on each side for about 10 minutes, or until golden brown and tender.

Meanwhile prepare sauce. In medium saucepan, cook green onion in butter until tender. Blend water with cornstarch and orange juice. Stir into sauce; cook for about 5 minutes, or until smooth and thickened. Add bouillon cubes, carrot, and orange peel. Cook on low heat for about 5 minutes (carrot should remain crunchy). Season with salt and pepper. Spoon over cooked turkey and serve.

MENU SUGGESTION

Skinless turkey breast is rich in protein but low in fat. Boost the fibre and vitamin A content of the meal and complement the colour, flavour, and texture of this dish with brown rice, peas, fresh sliced peaches, and low-fat milk. (Susan Close, R.P.Dt., Kitchener, Ontario)

Preparation: 20 minutes
Cook: 20 minutes
Makes 6 servings

Calories per serving: 444
Grams of protein per serving: 47.3
Grams of fat per serving: 11.5
Grams of carbohydrate per serving: 35.2
Grams of fibre per serving: 2.2

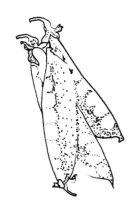

TURKIAKI FIESTA
Madeleine Dunbar-Maitland, Sudbury, Ontario

Ground turkey and chicken are becoming more readily available in supermarkets as an alternative to ground beef. This recipe utilizes either ground or slivered poultry with oriental seasonings and vegetables. Add extra teriyaki sauce if a stronger flavour is desired. Serve with cooked rice.

2 tsp.	vegetable oil	10 mL
1 lb.	ground or slivered turkey or chicken	500 g
2 tbsp.	teriyaki sauce	25 mL
Dash	salt and pepper	Dash
1 cup	diagonally sliced celery	250 mL
¾ cup	chopped green onions	175 mL
1	large red pepper, cubed	1
2 cups	snow peas, trimmed	500 mL
1	can (10 oz./284 mL) water chestnuts, drained	1
1 tbsp.	sesame seeds (optional)	15 mL

In wok or non-stick skillet, heat oil over high heat. Add turkey and stir-fry for about 4 minutes, or until lightly browned. Add teriyaki sauce, salt, pepper, celery, and onion. Cover and steam for 4 minutes. Add red pepper, snow peas, and water chestnuts; cover and cook for 6 minutes, stirring occasionally. Serve sprinkled with sesame seeds, if using.

MENU SUGGESTION
This entrée provides abundant high-quality protein with minimal fat. It is perfectly complemented by beef consommé aspic, brown rice, 2 percent milk, and tapioca pudding topped with fresh blueberries. (A. Harrison, R.P.Dt., Red Lake, Ontario)

Preparation: 10 minutes
Cook: about 10 minutes
Makes 4 to 5 servings

Calories per serving: 175
Grams of protein per serving: 23.1
Grams of fat per serving: 3.8
Grams of carbohydrate per serving: 11.8
Grams of fibre per serving: 3.8

Don't confuse cilantro with parsley. They look similar but they are different. Cilantro is the parsley-like leaf of the coriander plant. Cilantro leaves are more tender than parsley and have a zesty, almost bitter, flavour that lingers on the tongue. If you replace parsley with cilantro, do so carefully. You'll need less cilantro than parsley.

MENU SUGGESTION

Complement this dish with Rice Pilaf (page 160), and a colourful and crisp vegetable stir-fry of snow peas, red and yellow bell peppers, and mushrooms. Serve with a butter lettuce salad with mandarin orange sections and Raspberry Basil Vinaigrette (page 153). Complete the meal with fruit sorbet and milk. (Clinical Dietitians, Royal Columbian Hospital, New Westminster, British Columbia)

ORIENTAL FISH FILLETS
Joanne Rankin, Vancouver, British Columbia

This fabulous blend of exotic flavours results in fish-with-a-difference! Cilantro, commonly known as Chinese parsley, and gingerroot are responsible for the oriental flavouring.

4	green onions, diagonally sliced	4
2	cloves garlic, minced	2
1 tbsp.	canola oil	15 mL
4	fish fillets (turbot, cod, haddock, or halibut)	4
1 tbsp.	finely chopped gingerroot	15 mL
½ cup	dry sherry	125 mL
2 tbsp.	soy sauce	25 mL
¼ cup	coarsely chopped cilantro	50 mL

In heavy skillet on high heat, cook green onions and garlic in hot oil for about 2 minutes. Remove onion mixture and add fish to skillet.

Combine onion mixture, gingerroot, sherry, and soy sauce; pour over fish. Sprinkle with cilantro. Cook, covered, on medium heat for about 5 minutes, or until fish flakes easily with a fork. Remove fillets to preheated platter. Cook sauce on high heat until reduced and slightly thickened. Pour sauce over fish and serve.

Preparation: 10 minutes
Cook: about 8 minutes
Makes 4 servings

Calories per serving: 214
Grams of protein per serving: 25.3
Grams of fat per serving: 10.0
Grams of carbohydrate per serving: 4.8
Grams of fibre per serving: 0.5

CREAMY SALMON QUICHE
Joanne E. Yaraskavitch, Port Elgin, Ontario

This crustless quiche is prepared in a pie plate. An appetizer version of this recipe could be prepared in small tart tins.

¼ cup	dry, whole wheat bread crumbs	50 mL
1 tbsp.	all bran cereal, crushed	15 mL
1	can (7.5 oz./213 g) salmon	1
¼ cup	chopped green onion	50 mL
¼ cup	cubed light cream cheese	50 mL
1 tbsp.	chopped parsley	15 mL
1 ¼ cups	2 percent milk	300 mL
3	eggs	3
½ tsp.	white pepper	2 mL
	Paprika	

Combine bread crumbs and crushed cereal; sprinkle over bottom of non-stick or lightly greased pie plate.

Break salmon into chunks; arrange chunks over bread crumbs. Top with onion, cream cheese cubes, and parsley.

Whisk together milk, eggs, and pepper. Pour over salmon. Sprinkle lightly with paprika. Bake in 350°F (180°C) oven for 40 minutes, or until knife inserted in centre comes out clean. Allow to stand 5 minutes before cutting into wedges.

MENU SUGGESTION

This nutritious quiche is fairly high in fat, so serve it with low-fat accompaniments, such as Babsi's Broccoli Soup (page 59), tossed green salad with low-fat dressing, whole wheat rolls, and fresh fruit. The quiche and soup combine to provide almost one half the recommended daily intake of calcium for an adult. (Betty A. Brousse, R.P.Dt., Ottawa, Ontario)

Preparation: 10 minutes
Cook: 40 minutes
Makes 5 to 6 servings

Calories per serving: 153
Grams of protein per serving: 13.7
Grams of fat per serving: 7.6
Grams of carbohydrate per serving: 7.0
Grams of fibre per serving: 0.5

FISH ROLL-UPS
Pamela Najman, Downsview, Ontario

If you prefer, you can use frozen chopped spinach to replace fresh in this recipe. Just defrost one package and drain well. In combination with onions and mushrooms, the spinach is a pleasing filling for fish fillets.

½	package (10 oz./284 g) fresh spinach	½
1	small onion, chopped	1
1 tbsp.	butter or margarine	15 mL
1 cup	chopped mushrooms	250 mL
¼ cup	whole wheat bread crumbs	50 mL
1 lb.	sole fillets	500 g
	Salt, pepper, and thyme to taste	
½	lemon	½
	Garnish: paprika	

MENU SUGGESTION
This recipe is one of the lowest-fat entrées in the book. Complement the delicate blend of sole, spinach, and mushrooms with Mixed Rice Casserole (page 168) for fibre and texture and baby carrots for colour, and follow with sherbet and a melon slice. (Jane Hole, R.P.Dt., Hamilton, Ontario)

Steam spinach until tender; drain well.

In small skillet on medium-high heat, cook onion in butter for about 5 minutes, or until brown. Add mushrooms; cook 3 minutes.

In food processor, combine spinach, mushroom mixture, and bread crumbs. Process with on/off motion until coarsely chopped.

Season fish fillets with salt, pepper, and thyme. (If fish fillets are too wide, cut in half down centre of fillet.) Divide spinach filling over each fillet; roll up and secure with toothpicks. Place fish, seam side down, in non-stick or lightly greased baking pan. Squeeze lemon over fish; sprinkle with paprika. Bake, uncovered, in 425°F (220°C) oven for 10 minutes per inch (2.5 cm) of thickness, or until fish flakes easily with fork. Remove toothpicks and serve.

Preparation: 10 minutes
Cook: about 15 minutes
Makes 4 servings

Calories per serving: 144
Grams of protein per serving: 19.1
Grams of fat per serving: 4.1
Grams of carbohydrate per serving: 7.8
Grams of fibre per serving: 1.5

FISH FILLETS WITH BASIL WALNUT SAUCE

Betty Jane Humphrey, Owen Sound, Ontario

This easily prepared, marvellous sauce won the grand prize in The Canadian Dietetic Association Healthy Eating Recipe Contest. Similar to pesto, the sauce is quite thick, but may be thinned with chicken broth.

½ cup	fresh parsley, snipped and loosely packed	125 mL
½ cup	fresh basil, snipped and loosely packed	125 mL
3 tbsp.	finely chopped walnuts	45 mL
2 tbsp.	chicken broth	25 mL
2 tbsp.	grated Parmesan cheese	25 mL
1 tbsp.	olive oil	15 mL
1 tbsp.	balsamic vinegar or malt vinegar	15 mL
1 tsp.	granulated sugar	5 mL
1	clove garlic, minced	1
½ tsp.	freshly ground pepper	2 mL
1½ lb.	fish fillets (cod, haddock, or halibut) 1 inch (2.5 cm) thick	750 g
¼ cup	dry white wine	50 mL
½	lemon	½
1 tbsp.	butter or margarine	15 mL
	Salt and pepper to taste	

In food processor or blender, place parsley, basil, walnuts, chicken broth, cheese, oil, vinegar, sugar, garlic, and pepper. Process until smooth; add more broth if thinner sauce is desired.

Arrange fish in broiler or roasting pan. Pour wine into pan, squeeze lemon juice over fish. Dot with butter, sprinkle with salt and pepper. Broil 5 minutes. Spoon sauce over and broil another 4 to 5 minutes, allowing total of 10 minutes per inch (2.5 cm) of thickness.

MENU SUGGESTION

High-fibre brown rice will complement this dish with its marvellous sauce of fresh herbs, cheese, and walnuts. The walnuts and oil in the recipe contribute fat, so keep the accompanying dishes low in fat. Add mixed vegetables and tomato slices on greens with low-cal dressing for contrasting colours and textures. Finish the meal with low-fat peach yoghurt. (Susan Close, R.P.Dt., Kitchener, Ontario)

Preparation: 10 minutes
Cook: 10 minutes
Makes 6 servings

Calories per serving: 200
Grams of protein per serving: 24.8
Grams of fat per serving: 9.4
Grams of carbohydrate per serving: 3.2
Grams of fibre per serving: 0.4

BARBECUED STUFFED SALMON
Maureen Prairie, Thunder Bay, Ontario

To cook fish on the barbecue, put it in a fish cooker or wrap it loosely in foil left open at the top. This way the fish will remain moist, yet have that great barbecue flavour.

1	small onion, finely chopped	1
2	cloves garlic, minced	2
1	stalk celery, finely chopped	1
1 tbsp.	butter or margarine	15 mL
1	can (4 ½ oz./128 g) crab meat, drained	1
1 cup	cooked rice	250 mL
2 tbsp.	lemon juice	25 mL
1 tbsp.	finely chopped parsley	15 mL
1 tsp.	grated lemon peel	5 mL
½ tsp.	salt	2 mL
¼ tsp.	pepper	1 mL
2	salmon fillets (1 ½ lb./750 g)	2
½	lemon, sliced	½

In medium skillet on high heat, cook onion, garlic, and celery in butter until softened. Stir in crab meat, rice, lemon juice, parsley, lemon peel, and seasonings.

Place stuffing over one fish fillet; top with second fillet. Secure with string or toothpicks. Arrange lemon slices on top. Wrap loosely in several thicknesses of aluminum foil.

Place on barbecue grill. Cook for about 45 minutes, or until fish flakes easily with fork, or bake in 450°F (230°C) oven for 10 minutes per inch (2.5 cm) of thickness.

MENU SUGGESTION

This quick and simple dish is perfect for summer entertaining. It contributes protein and B vitamins. Serve with whole wheat pita bread and spinach salad with Sesame Vinaigrette (page 154) for extra fibre, followed by Strawberry Sorbet (page 223). (Kelly McQuillen, Whitehorse, Yukon)

Preparation: 15 minutes
Cook: 45 minutes
Makes 6 servings

Calories per serving: 238
Grams of protein per serving: 28.5
Grams of fat per serving: 9.1
Grams of carbohydrate per serving: 8.7
Grams of fibre per serving: 0.4

Photos: Cottage Cheese-Filled Crepes, page 101 (facing page); Falafel, page 111, and Tabbouleh, page 150 (overleaf)

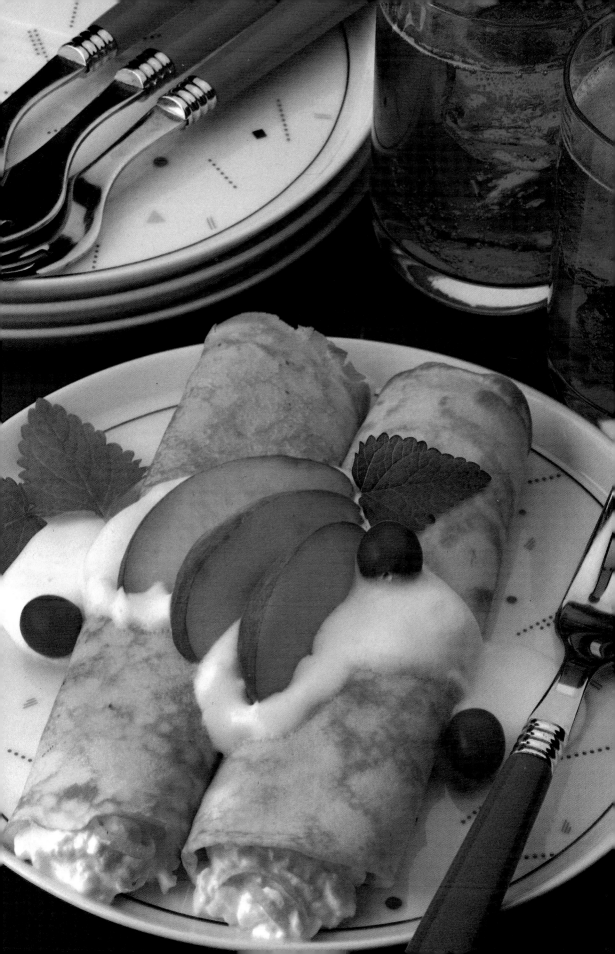

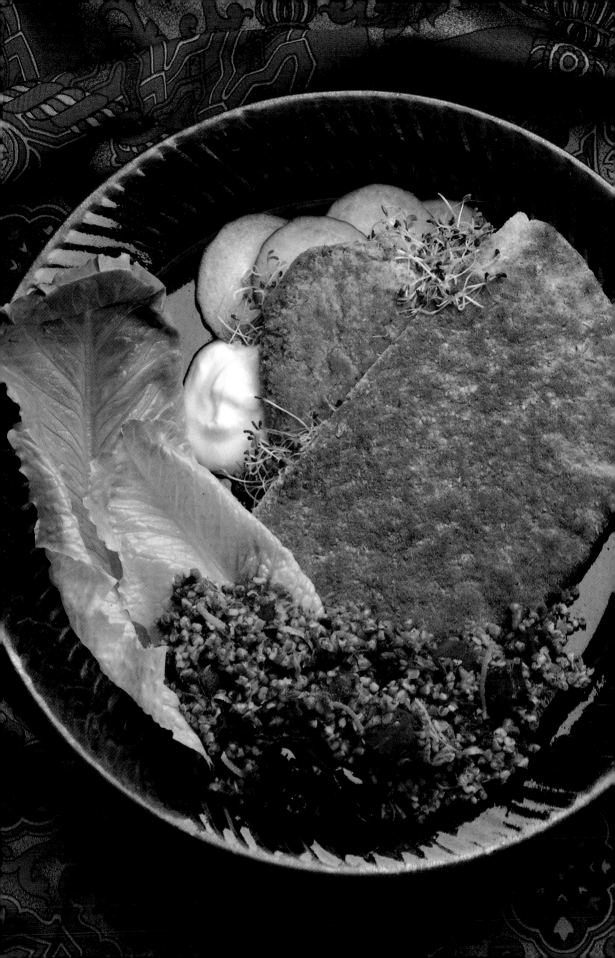

CHEESY SALMON LOAF
Claire Lightfoot, Campbell River, British Columbia

Grated carrot provides a new interest to this basic salmon loaf. The whole family will love it.

MENU SUGGESTION
This recipe provides generous amounts of high-quality protein, niacin, vitamin A, and calcium. Add Rice Pilaf (page 160) for fibre. Served with steamed asparagus with calorie-reduced vinaigrette and a multigrain roll, followed by Fruit with Yoghurt Dressing (page 212), you have a nutritionally superior meal. (Rosario Soneff, R.D.N., Penticton, British Columbia)

2	eggs	2
1 cup	rolled oats	250 mL
2	cans (each 7.5 oz./213 g) salmon	2
1 cup	grated low-fat mozzarella cheese	250 mL
¼ cup	chopped onion	50 mL
1	stalk celery, chopped	1
1	large carrot, grated	1
2 tbsp.	lemon juice	25 mL

In large bowl, beat eggs. Stir in rolled oats, salmon, cheese, onion, celery, carrot, and lemon juice until well combined. Turn salmon mixture into non-stick or lightly greased 9 × 5-inch (2 L) loaf pan. Bake in 350°F (180°C) oven for about 35 minutes. Allow to stand 5 minutes before slicing.

Preparation: 10 minutes
Cook: about 35 minutes
Makes 6 servings

Calories per serving: 235
Grams of protein per serving: 23.6
Grams of fat per serving: 10.0
Grams of carbohydrate per serving: 11.6
Grams of fibre per serving: 1.8

SAUCE

1 cup	orange juice	250 mL
¼ cup	water	50 mL
2 tbsp.	cornstarch	25 mL
2 tbsp.	liquid honey	25 mL
1 tsp.	grated orange peel	5 mL
1 tsp.	grated lemon peel	5 mL
1 tsp.	Dijon mustard	5 mL
1 cup	fresh orange sections	250 mL
1 cup	seedless green grapes, halved	250 mL
	Garnish: mint leaves	

MENU SUGGESTION

Serve this low-fat dish with brown rice and spinach salad to increase the fibre and iron content of the meal. Finish the meal with fresh fruit for a delicious low-fat way to eat from Canada's Food Guide. (MaryAnne Zupancic, R.D.N., Nanaimo, British Columbia)

Preparation: 10 minutes
Cook: 8 to 10 minutes
Makes 6 servings

Calories per serving: 161
Grams of protein per serving: 17.2
Grams of fat per serving: 1.1
Grams of carbohydrate per serving: 21.1
Grams of fibre per serving: 1.1

GRAPE AND ORANGE SOLE SUPREME
Fran J. Maki, Surrey, British Columbia

This colourful fish recipe needs only rice and either a vegetable or a salad to turn it into a complete meal. You can substitute halibut, haddock, or turbot for sole.

1½ lb.	sole fillets	750 g
1½ cups	boiling water	375 mL
⅓ cup	finely chopped onion	75 mL
2 tbsp.	lemon juice	25 mL
¾ tsp.	salt	4 mL

Roll fish fillets and secure with toothpicks. Arrange in shallow skillet. Add boiling water, onion, lemon juice, and salt. Poach, covered, on low heat for about 8 minutes.

To microwave, place fish in casserole, omit water but sprinkle fish with lemon juice and salt, cover. Microwave on High (100 percent), for 5 to 7 minutes, or until fish flakes easily with a fork.

Meanwhile, prepare sauce. In small saucepan, combine orange juice, water, cornstarch, honey, orange and lemon peel, and mustard. Cook over low heat, stirring constantly until thickened. Add orange sections and green grapes.

Spoon sauce over drained fish fillets and garnish with mint leaves.

ORIENTAL SEAFOOD FONDUE
Diana Sheh, Toronto, Ontario

Oriental fondue is a lower-fat version, using chicken broth rather than oil to cook the seafood, tofu, and vegetables. After these items have been eaten, the remaining delicious broth can be served as a soup course.

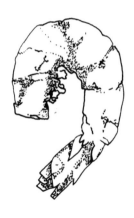

2½ cups	chicken broth	625 mL
¼ cup	chopped fresh cilantro	50 mL
1 tbsp.	chopped gingerroot	15 mL
1	small clove garlic, minced	1
¼ tsp.	cayenne pepper	1 mL
1 lb.	seafood (scallops, shrimp, lobster tails, cut into bite-sized pieces)	500 g
12	small whole mushrooms	12
½ lb.	firm tofu, drained, cut into bite-sized pieces	250 g
6	green onions, cut into 2-inch (5 cm) pieces	6
2 cups	spinach leaves, trimmed	500 mL
	Cooked white rice (approximately 3 cups/750 mL)	
	Dipping sauces: Oriental sweet and sour or plum sauce (available in most grocery stores)	
1 cup	finely shredded cabbage	250 mL

Preparation: 20 minutes
Cook: about 10 minutes
Makes 6 to 8 servings

Calories per serving: 113
Grams of protein per serving: 15.6
Grams of fat per serving: 4.0
Grams of carbohydrate per serving: 5.1
Grams of fibre per serving: 1.2

In fondue pot, heat chicken broth, cilantro, gingerroot, garlic, and cayenne pepper to boiling.

Arrange seafood, mushrooms, tofu, white part of onion, and spinach on large platter. Using fondue fork, dip pieces of seafood, tofu, and vegetables into hot broth, cooking to desired doneness. Serve with rice and dipping sauces.

When all seafood and vegetables have been cooked, add cabbage and green part of onion to broth; cook for several minutes. Serve soup in individual bowls.

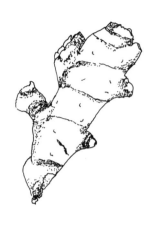

GINGER VEGETABLE-BEEF MEDLEY

Maisie S. Vanriel, Toronto, Ontario

Vegetables can be varied in this beef stir-fry—red or white onions, sliced carrots, snow peas, chopped broccoli, or cauliflower. Remember that brown rice is not only more flavourful than white, it is also more nutritious. Be sure to try it in this recipe.

1½ cups	brown rice	375 mL
4 cups	boiling water	1 L
¼ cup	safflower oil, divided	50 mL
2	small onions, cut into wedges	2
1	clove garlic, minced	1
½ lb.	green beans, diagonally sliced	250 g
1 lb.	mushrooms, sliced	500 g
1 cup	sliced water chestnuts	250 mL
2 tsp.	chopped gingerroot	10 mL
½ tsp.	black pepper	2 mL
1½ lb.	sirloin or top round steak, cut into thin strips	750 g
3 tbsp.	cornstarch	45 mL
2 tsp.	ground ginger	10 mL
½ cup	water	125 mL
⅓ cup	chili sauce	75 mL
¼ cup	soy sauce	50 mL

In saucepan, add rice to boiling water. Cover and cook 45 minutes, or until tender and water is absorbed.

In wok or non-stick skillet, heat 2 tbsp. (25 mL) oil over high heat. Add onions and garlic; stir-fry for 1 minute. Add green beans, mushrooms, and water chestnuts. Cover and steam for 4 minutes. Stir in gingerroot and pepper. Remove mixture and keep warm.

Coat beef strips in cornstarch and ginger. In wok, stir-fry beef on high heat in remaining oil until brown. Stir in water, chili sauce, and soy sauce.

Arrange rice on platter; top with vegetable mixture and beef strips.

MENU SUGGESTION

This hearty dish is almost a meal in itself, as it is loaded with high-quality protein, B vitamins, iron, and fibre. For light accompaniments to the meal, start with mulligatawny soup and finish with Lemon Pudding (page 232). (Patti Benzer, R.D.N., Kelowna, British Columbia)

Preparation: 45 minutes
Cook: about 10 minutes
Makes 6 servings

Calories per serving: 552
Grams of protein per serving: 31.2
Grams of fat per serving: 19.7
Grams of carbohydrate per serving: 62.8
Grams of fibre per serving: 5.3

CURRIED BEEF CUBES
Judith Halladay, Whitby, Ontario.

This quick-cooking curry is perfect for an everyday meal or for a buffet casserole at a party. Freeze the sauce and reheat it in either the microwave or the oven to serve over rice or noodles.

MENU SUGGESTION

Serve this recipe with rice or noodles and cucumber strips with yoghurt for a main course rich in protein, iron, and B vitamins. Boost the fibre content by using brown rice. Finish the meal with the spicy taste of Hot Water Gingerbread (page 233). (Laurie Daniels, R.P.Dt., London, Ontario)

1 lb.	stewing beef, cubed	500 g
1	medium Spanish onion, sliced	1
1 tbsp.	butter or margarine	15 mL
1	can (19 oz./540 mL) tomatoes	1
3 tbsp.	desiccated coconut or	45 mL
⅓ cup	raisins	75 mL
1 tbsp.	lemon juice	15 mL
1 tsp.	granulated sugar	5 mL
1 tsp.	chili powder	5 mL
1 tsp.	ground turmeric	5 mL
½ tsp.	curry powder	2 mL
½ tsp.	salt	2 mL
¼ tsp.	ground cinnamon	1 mL
Dash	ground cloves	Dash

Preparation: 20 minutes
Cook: 1 to 2 hours
Makes 4 to 5 servings

Calories per serving with coconut: 208
Grams of protein per serving: 20.0
Grams of fat per serving: 8.9
Grams of carbohydrate per serving: 11.7
Grams of fibre per serving: 2.6

Calories per serving with raisins: 222
Grams of protein per serving: 20.3
Grams of fat per serving: 7.7
Grams of carbohydrate per serving: 18.4
Grams of fibre per serving: 2.3

In large Dutch oven or stockpot over medium-high heat, brown beef and onion in butter for about 10 minutes. Add tomatoes, coconut, lemon juice, sugar, and seasonings. Cook, covered, on low heat for about 2 hours, or until meat is tender. Taste and add extra curry powder if required. Serve over cooked rice or noodles.

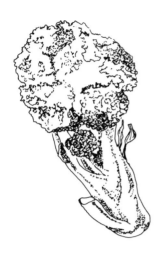

BEEF WITH BROCCOLI
M. Kathy Dyck, Weyburn, Saskatchewan

This recipe provides a marriage of oriental flavours, and is best served with cooked white or brown rice.

1 lb.	sirloin steak, cut into thin strips	500 g
¼ cup	soy sauce	50 mL
2 tbsp.	cornstarch, divided	25 mL
1	clove garlic, minced	1
1	thin slice gingerroot, minced	1
2 tbsp.	safflower oil, divided	25 mL
2	medium onions, cut into wedges	2
3	large carrots, sliced into coins	3
1	head broccoli, cut into florets	1
1¼ cups	water, divided	300 mL
1 tbsp.	oyster sauce	15 mL
1 tbsp.	cornstarch	15 mL
1 tsp.	granulated sugar	5 mL

Place steak in medium bowl. In separate bowl, combine soy sauce, 1 tbsp. (15 mL) cornstarch, garlic, and gingerroot; pour over meat.

In wok or non-stick skillet, heat 1 tbsp. (15 mL) oil over high heat. Add beef and stir-fry until meat is brown. Set aside.

In wok, heat remaining oil over high heat. Add onions and stir-fry for 1 minute. Add carrots, broccoli, and 1 cup (250 mL) water. Cover and steam for 4 minutes.

Combine remaining water, oyster sauce, 1 tbsp. (15 mL) cornstarch, and sugar. Stir sauce into wok; cook, until smooth and thickened. Return meat to wok. Reheat to serving temperature. Serve over cooked rice.

MENU SUGGESTION

Since the oil used in stir-frying contributes a significant proportion of the fat to this dish, balance the meal with accompaniments that have minimal fat content. For a delightful meal with an oriental theme, begin with consommé, and serve the main course with mixed Chinese vegetables and brown rice. Follow with Chinese melon and lychee nuts which contribute complex carbohydrates and fibre. (Merry Ellis, P.Dt., Regina, Saskatchewan)

Preparation: 15 minutes
Cook: about 10 minutes
Makes 4 to 6 servings

Calories per serving: 189
Grams of protein per serving: 14.7
Grams of fat per serving: 9.6
Grams of carbohydrate per serving: 11.4
Grams of fibre per serving: 2.1

CONFETTI PORK

Marilyn Grisé, Saskatoon, Saskatchewan

One of the delights of stir-fried vegetables is their crunchy texture and bright colour. As well, vegetables retain nutrients better when cooked by this method.

MENU SUGGESTION

This dish contains ingredients from three food groups as well as a hefty dose of iron. Serve it with mixed greens with Raspberry Basil Vinaigrette (page 153) and whole wheat dinner rolls. Finish the meal with dairy-rich baked custard with lemon sauce. (Marilyn Grisé, P.Dt., Saskatoon, Saskatchewan)

1 lb.	pork tenderloin, cut into thin strips	500 g
¼ cup	teriyaki sauce	50 mL
1 cup	water	250 mL
½ cup	dried apricots, halved	125 mL
2 ½ cups	pineapple or orange juice	625 mL
1 ¼ cups	white rice	300 mL
1 tbsp.	vegetable oil	15 mL
1	medium onion, chopped	1
1	medium red pepper, chopped	1
1	small yellow pepper, chopped	1
¼ cup	slivered almonds	50 mL

Marinate pork in teriyaki sauce for several hours in refrigerator.

Bring water and apricots to boil in small saucepan. Cook for about 20 minutes, or until tender. Remove apricots, reserve liquid. Add pineapple juice to saucepan; return to boil, add rice and cook for about 15 minutes, or until rice is tender and liquid is absorbed.

In large skillet, on medium-high heat, stir-fry pork in hot oil for about 5 minutes, or until browned. Add onion and peppers; stir-fry for 5 minutes. Stir in apricots and almonds. Serve over rice.

Preparation: 20 minutes
Marinate: several hours
Cook: 20 minutes
Makes 4 to 5 servings

Calories per serving: 471
Grams of protein per serving: 26.7
Grams of fat per serving: 9.8
Grams of carbohydrate per serving: 68.8
Grams of fibre per serving: 3.7

CURRIED LAMB CHOPS
Carol Oldford, Moncton, New Brunswick

Experiment with herbs in your cooking to give a quick and subtle change to your recipes. Rosemary is generally used with lamb, but try curry and enjoy the difference.

MENU SUGGESTION

Combined with vegetables and a light dessert, this meal will not only satisfy the palate but will also provide a good source of vitamins, calcium, and iron. Serve with Blond Sangria (page 238), Spaghetti Squash (page 130), and Dilly Bread (page 186), followed by mint gelatine dessert with low-fat yoghurt. (Elizabeth Farrell, P.Dt., Saint John, New Brunswick)

6	loin lamb chops, 1½-inch (4 cm) thick	6
2 tbsp.	white wine vinegar	25 mL
1 tsp.	salt	5 mL
¼ tsp.	pepper	1 mL
2 tsp.	vegetable oil	10 mL
1 tsp.	curry powder	5 mL
1 tsp.	finely chopped gingerroot	5 mL
1	clove garlic, minced	1
¼ tsp.	ground cloves	1 mL
¼ tsp.	ground cinnamon	1 mL
¾ cup	water, divided	175 mL
1	medium onion, chopped	1
2 tbsp.	all-purpose flour	25 mL
2 tbsp.	currants	25 mL
1	kiwi fruit, peeled and sliced	1
1	orange, peeled and sliced	1

Place lamb chops in shallow pan. Combine vinegar, salt, and pepper. Spoon over chops. Set aside for 5 minutes.

In heavy skillet, cook oil, curry, gingerroot, garlic, and seasonings until mixture bubbles. Add ½ cup (125 mL) water and onion. Cook over medium heat for about 5 minutes.

Sprinkle flour over lamb chops; add chops to onions in skillet. Cook about 4 minutes per side, or until chops lose pink colour. Stir in remaining water and currants. Cook, covered, over low heat for about 30 minutes, or until chops are tender. Add kiwi fruit and oranges and cook for about 3 minutes.

Preparation: 15 minutes
Cook: 35 minutes
Makes 6 servings

Calories per serving: 217
Grams of protein per serving: 24.9
Grams of fat per serving: 8.0
Grams of carbohydrate per serving: 10.6
Grams of fibre per serving: 1.2

APPLE ROSEMARY MARINADE

¾ cup	unsweetened frozen concentrated apple juice, thawed	175 mL
½ cup	cider vinegar	125 mL
¼ cup	liquid honey	50 mL
1 tbsp.	soy sauce	15 mL
1 tsp.	dried rosemary	5 mL

Makes about 1 ½ cups (375 mL)

GINGER YOGHURT MARINADE

1 cup	low-fat plain yoghurt	250 mL
1 tbsp.	minced gingerroot	15 mL
2 tsp.	ground coriander	10 mL
1 tsp.	grated orange rind	5 mL
¼ tsp.	hot pepper sauce	1 mL

Makes about 1 cup (250 mL)

LEMON PESTO MARINADE

½ cup	chicken broth	125 mL
2 tbsp.	Lemon Pesto Sauce (page 177)	25 mL
2 tbsp.	white wine vinegar	25 mL

Makes ¾ cup (175 mL)

Preparation: 5 minutes
Marinate: 8 hours or overnight

MARINADES FOR MEAT
Janine MacLachlan, Toronto, Ontario

Try one of the following delicious marinades with the meat of your choice. They are all lower in fat than traditional marinades.

Apple Rosemary Marinade for lamb, or pork

Ginger Yoghurt Marinade for poultry, or pork

Lemon Pesto for chicken, fish, veal, or lamb

Sherry Lemon Marinade for lamb, chicken, beef, or pork

Beer Carbonara for lamb, beef or pork

Each of these recipes makes sufficient marinade for up to 3 lbs. (1.5 kg) meat.

To prepare, combine ingredients for the chosen marinade (see above). Place meat in plastic bag or shallow pan; pour marinade over meat. Refrigerate 8 hours or overnight, turning meat once or twice. Just before cooking, drain meat, reserving marinade; use the reserved marinade to brush meat during cooking.

SHERRY LEMON MARINADE

½ cup	dry sherry	125 mL
2	cloves garlic, crushed	2
2 tbsp.	soy sauce	25 mL
2 tbsp.	lemon juice	25 mL
1 tbsp.	dried tarragon	15 mL
1 tsp.	grated lemon rind	5 mL
	Freshly ground pepper	

Makes about 1 cup (250 mL)

BEER CARBONARA MARINADE

1 cup	beer	250 mL
½ cup	chopped onions	125 mL
2 tbsp.	vegetable oil	25 mL
2 tsp.	brown sugar	10 mL
2 tsp.	Dijon mustard	10 mL
	Freshly ground pepper to taste	

Makes about 1 cup (250 mL).

ZESTY HERB STUFFING
The Canadian Dietetic Association, Toronto, Ontario

A simple and tasty idea to add a gourmet touch to fish and poultry. Lime or lemon juice may be replaced with tomato juice and a dash of hot pepper sauce. Be creative and experiment with the ingredients. Try shredded carrot, raisins, chopped tomato, grape halves, crushed pineapple, apple chunks and so on. As well, other herbs and seasonings may be used, especially if using dry bread crumbs.

1	stalk celery, finely chopped	1
½	medium onion, finely chopped	½
1 cup	seasoned croutons, crushed or	250 mL
½ cup	dry bread crumbs	125 mL
2 tbsp.	lemon or lime juice	25 mL
¼ tsp.	pepper	1 mL
	Fish fillets or boneless chicken breasts	

Combine celery, onion, croutons or crumbs, lemon juice, and pepper. Place several spoonfuls on either a fish fillet or chicken breast. Roll up; secure with toothpick, and bake covered in 425°F (220°C) oven (for fish) or in 350°F (180°C) oven (for chicken). Allow 10 minutes per inch (2.5 cm) of thickness for fish.

Makes 4 servings

Calories per serving: 53
Grams of protein per serving: 1.7
Grams of fat per serving: 0.6
Grams of carbohydrate per serving: 10.5
Grams of fibre per serving: 0.8

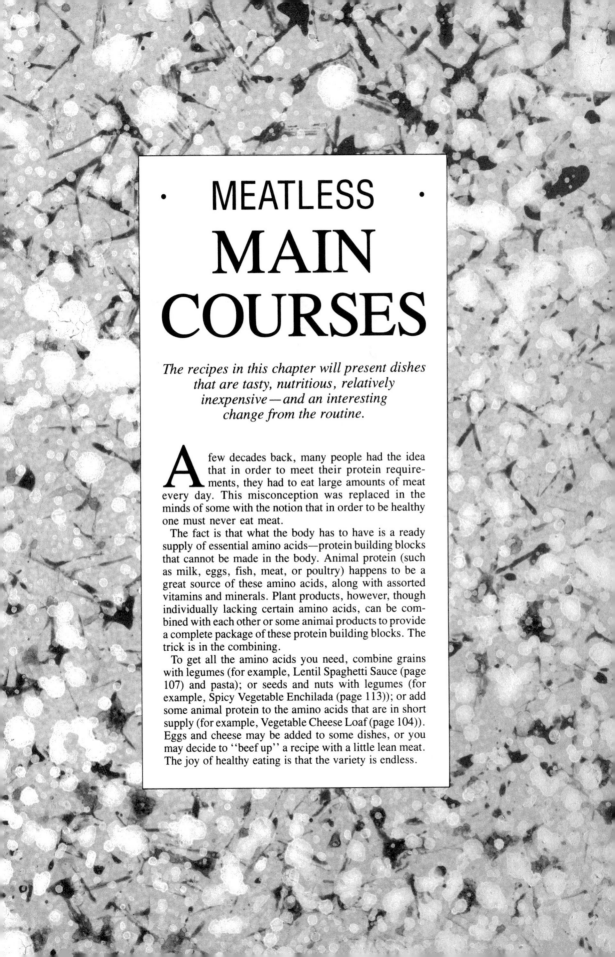

· MEATLESS
MAIN
COURSES

*The recipes in this chapter will present dishes
that are tasty, nutritious, relatively
inexpensive—and an interesting
change from the routine.*

A few decades back, many people had the idea
that in order to meet their protein require-
ments, they had to eat large amounts of meat
every day. This misconception was replaced in the
minds of some with the notion that in order to be healthy
one must never eat meat.

The fact is that what the body has to have is a ready
supply of essential amino acids—protein building blocks
that cannot be made in the body. Animal protein (such
as milk, eggs, fish, meat, or poultry) happens to be a
great source of these amino acids, along with assorted
vitamins and minerals. Plant products, however, though
individually lacking certain amino acids, can be combined with each other or some animal products to provide
a complete package of these protein building blocks. The
trick is in the combining.

To get all the amino acids you need, combine grains
with legumes (for example, Lentil Spaghetti Sauce (page
107) and pasta); or seeds and nuts with legumes (for
example, Spicy Vegetable Enchilada (page 113)); or add
some animal protein to the amino acids that are in short
supply (for example, Vegetable Cheese Loaf (page 104)).
Eggs and cheese may be added to some dishes, or you
may decide to ''beef up'' a recipe with a little lean meat.
The joy of healthy eating is that the variety is endless.

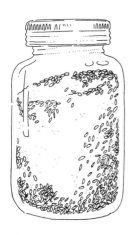

MAGIC MEATLESS CASSEROLE
Donalda Murray, Cornwall, Ontario

Since brown rice requires about 45 minutes cooking time, it is a good idea to cook a larger amount than you require and freeze it for recipes like this one. Voilà, this side-dish can be ready in minutes instead of one hour.

1 cup	brown rice	250 mL
3¾ cups	water, divided	925 mL
1 cup	sliced celery	250 mL
½ cup	chopped onion	125 mL
2 tbsp.	vegetable oil	25 mL
1	can (19 oz./540 mL) tomatoes	1
⅔ cup	chopped ripe olives	150 mL
2 tbsp.	all-purpose flour	25 mL
2 tsp.	chili powder	10 mL
1 tsp.	salt	5 mL
¼ tsp.	garlic powder	1 mL
1 cup	frozen peas	250 mL
⅔ cup	shredded Cheddar cheese	150 mL

In saucepan, bring 3 cups (750 mL) water to boil. Add rice. Cook, covered, for 45 minutes, or until rice is tender and water is absorbed.

Meanwhile, in medium saucepan on high heat, cook celery and onion in oil for about 5 minutes, or until tender. Add tomatoes and olives; bring to boil. Mix flour, seasonings, and remaining water; stir into hot mixture. Cook for about 3 minutes, or until thickened. Stir in frozen peas.

Pour half sauce mixture into an 8-cup (2-L) casserole. Top with cooked rice and remaining sauce. Sprinkle with cheese. Bake at 350°F (180°C) for about 20 minutes, or until heated through.

MENU SUGGESTION

Serve this high-fibre recipe with devilled eggs to provide an additional source of protein for the cheese in the casserole. A tossed green salad, whole wheat rolls, and a fresh fruit salad complete the meal. (Audrey Shackleton, P.Dt., Bathurst, New Brunswick)

Preparation: 45 minutes
Cook: 25 minutes
Makes 6 servings

Calories per serving: 294
Grams of protein per serving: 8.6
Grams of fat per serving: 11.8
Grams of carbohydrate per serving: 39.7
Grams of fibre per serving: 4.6

COTTAGE CHEESE-FILLED CRÊPES
Teresa Feduszczak, Vinemount, Ontario

These crêpes are similar to cheese blintzes. Serve for brunch or lunch with fresh fruit and yoghurt, or as a dessert. You can substitute dry-curd or pressed cottage cheese to achieve a drier filling. For extra protein, increase the amount of cottage cheese filling in each crêpe.

FILLING

1 cup	creamed low-fat (2 percent) cottage cheese, drained, or pressed cottage cheese	250 mL
1	egg, lightly beaten	1
2 tbsp.	granulated sugar	25 mL
¼ tsp.	vanilla extract	1 mL
½ tsp.	grated lemon rind	2 mL
1 tbsp.	butter or margarine	15 mL

CRÊPE

½ cup	all-purpose flour	125 mL
1 tbsp.	granulated sugar	15 mL
½ tsp.	salt	2 mL
2	eggs	2
⅔ cup	2 percent milk	150 mL

Combine flour, sugar, and salt. Beat eggs until light and fluffy. Add milk; mix well. Add dry ingredients to egg mixture, beat with rotary or hand mixer until smooth. Allow mixture to rest for 30 minutes to 1 hour.

Heat non-stick 8-inch (20 cm) crêpe or omelet pan. Pour about ¼ cup (50 mL) batter into pan. When bottom looks done, loosen and flip. (This is a test crêpe). When pan is ready, pour ¼ cup (50 mL) batter into pan; swirl until bottom is coated. Cook until crêpe is brown, then flip out of pan cooking only one side. Repeat with remaining batter.

In medium bowl, combine cottage cheese, beaten egg, sugar, vanilla, and lemon rind. Spread filling evenly over uncooked side of each crêpe. Roll up crêpes; place seam-side down in non-stick or lightly greased oven-proof baking dish. Dot each crêpe with butter. Cover and bake in 300°F (150°C) oven for about 20 minutes.

MENU SUGGESTION

These crêpes are rich in protein and low in fat and calories. Serve them with carrots and a fresh garden salad to provide extra vitamins and fibre. Finish the meal with a fruit compote or low-fat fruit sorbet. (Dianne M. Johns, P.Dt., Saskatoon, Saskatchewan)

Preparation: 15 minutes
Cook: 10 minutes
Makes 8 crêpes

Calories per crêpe: 121
Grams of protein per crêpe: 7.1
Grams of fat per crêpe: 4.4
Grams of carbohydrate per crêpe: 12.8
Grams of fibre per crêpe: 0.2

MEXICAN PIE
Barbara Silvester, Moosomin, Saskatchewan

Prepare this recipe ahead and freeze or refrigerate for apres-ski or a busy Saturday evening meal. For a spicier flavour, increase the amount of chili powder.

1	medium onion, chopped	1
1 tbsp.	vegetable oil	15 mL
1	can (19 oz./540 mL) tomatoes	1
1	can (14 oz./398 mL) kidney beans	1
1	can (12 oz./341 mL) whole kernel corn	1
1 tbsp.	chili powder	15 mL
¾ cup	cornmeal	175 mL
1 cup	2 percent milk	250 mL
2	eggs	2
1½ cups	shredded cheese (old Cheddar, Swiss, mozzarella or a mixture of all three)	375 mL

In large skillet on medium-high heat, cook onion in oil until transparent. Cut up tomatoes. Add tomatoes, kidney beans, corn, and chili powder to skillet. Cook on low heat, uncovered, for about 1 hour, or until slightly thickened; stir occasionally. Pour mixture into 9 × 13-inch (3.5 L) baking pan. Sprinkle cornmeal evenly over surface.

In separate bowl, beat together milk and eggs; pour evenly over cornmeal. Sprinkle with cheese. Bake in 350°F (180°C) oven for 50 to 55 minutes. Cut into squares to serve.

MENU SUGGESTION

The beans, cornmeal, cheese, milk, and eggs in this vegetarian recipe combine to provide top-quality protein. To add extra fibre, serve with a spinach salad with Sesame Vinaigrette (page 154) and a multi-grain roll. Blond Sangria (page 238) and winter fruit compote with figs and apricots complete a meal that is a great source of calcium, iron, vitamin A, and vitamin C. (Elaine Power, R.Dt., Port aux Basques, Newfoundland)

Preparation: 1 hour
Cook: 50 minutes
Makes 6 servings

Calories per serving: 350
Grams of protein per serving: 17.6
Grams of fat per serving: 13.8
Grams of carbohydrate per serving: 41.6
Grams of fibre per serving: 6.9

VEGETABLE LOVER'S CHILI
Laura M. Hawthorn, Bracebridge, Ontario

This wonderful chili recipe makes a very large quantity—about 12 servings—but you can always freeze any leftovers.

MENU SUGGESTION

Serve this hearty, high-fibre dish with fresh corn bread to complement the protein from the beans in the chili, and add mixed garden greens with low-cal dressing for additional vitamins. Lemon sorbet with blueberry purée topping for dessert is a refreshing contrast to the spicy chili. (Monica Beck, P.Dt., Halifax, Nova Scotia)

2	cans (each 28 oz./796 mL) tomatoes	2
2	cans (each 14 oz./398 mL) kidney beans, drained	2
2 cups	chopped celery	500 mL
2 cups	chopped carrots	500 mL
1 cup	chopped onion	250 mL
½ cup	chopped green pepper	125 mL
½ cup	raisins	125 mL
¼ cup	cider vinegar	50 mL
1 tbsp.	chili powder	15 mL
1 tbsp.	dried parsley flakes	15 mL
1½ tsp.	dried oregano	7 mL
1 tsp.	salt	5 mL
1 tsp.	ground allspice	5 mL
½ tsp.	dried basil	2 mL
¼ tsp.	hot pepper sauce	1 mL
1 cup	light beer	250 mL
1 cup	shredded old Cheddar cheese	250 mL
	Garnish: crushed corn flakes	

Preparation: 20 minutes
Cook: 1½ hours
Makes 12 servings.

Calories per serving: 167
Grams of protein per serving: 8.1
Grams of fat per serving: 3.9
Grams of carbohydrate per serving: 26.4
Grams of fibre per serving: 6.9

In large stockpot, combine tomatoes, kidney beans, celery, carrots, onion, green pepper, raisins, vinegar, and seasonings. Cover and cook for about 30 minutes. Uncover and cook for another 30 minutes. Stir in the beer. Simmer, uncovered, for about 25 minutes, or until thickened. Serve garnished with cheese and crushed corn flakes.

VEGETABLE CHEESE LOAF WITH LEMON TOMATO SAUCE
Margaret McIntyre, Woodstock, Ontario

Unusual but very tasty! Serve this appetizing vegetarian loaf as a main course at brunch or dinner. With the refreshing tang of lemon in the loaf and in the Lemon Tomato Sauce, this recipe will easily become a favourite.

¾ cup	finely chopped onion	175 mL
3 tbsp.	butter or margarine	45 mL
¾ cup	finely chopped celery	175 mL
2	medium carrots, peeled and grated	2
2 cups	small-curd cottage cheese	500 mL
2 cups	fresh bread crumbs	500 mL
2	eggs, well beaten	2
½	lemon rind and juice	½
1 tsp.	salt	5 mL
½ tsp.	pepper	2 mL
¼ tsp.	dried basil	1 mL

In medium skillet on medium heat, cook onion in melted butter for about 5 minutes, or until tender. Add celery and carrots; cook 1 minute.

In large bowl, combine cottage cheese, bread crumbs, eggs, lemon rind and juice, and seasonings. Add vegetable mixture; stir.

Place in non-stick or lightly greased 9 × 5-inch (2 L) baking pan. Bake in 350°F (180°C) oven for 35 to 40 minutes or until knife inserted in centre comes out clean. Remove loaf from pan.

To make sauce: in medium saucepan, combine 1½ cups (375 mL) tomato juice, onion, parsley, seasonings, and sugar. Bring to boil, reduce heat, and simmer for 15 to 20 minutes. Press mixture through sieve. Reserve sieved tomato mixture.

In small saucepan, melt butter and blend in flour; cook 1 to 2 minutes. Gradually add remaining tomato juice. Cook, stirring constantly for 4 to 5 minutes, or until smooth and thickened. Add reserved tomato mixture and lemon juice. Reheat to serving temperature.

To serve, slice loaf, pour sauce over slices.

SAUCE

2½ cups	tomato juice, divided	625 mL
1	medium onion, cut in half	1
4	parsley sprigs	4
1	bay leaf	1
1	whole clove	1
½ tsp.	dried basil	2 mL
½ tsp.	granulated sugar	2 mL
⅓ cup	butter or margarine	75 mL
¼ cup	all-purpose flour	50 mL
½	lemon, squeezed	½

MENU SUGGESTION

Use the lemon tomato sauce sparingly in this recipe to minimize fat and calories. Add fibre to the meal with Babsi's Broccoli Soup (page 59), Carrot Bran Muffins (page 191), and whole wheat crêpes with raspberry sauce. (Patti Benzer, R.D.N., Kelowna, British Columbia)

Preparation: 30 minutes
Cook: 35 to 40 minutes
Makes 6 servings

Calories per serving: 319
Grams of protein per serving: 15.1
Grams of fat per serving: 19.2
Grams of carbohydrate per serving: 22.8
Grams of fibre per serving: 1.5

ZUCCHINI FRITTATA
Ruth Borthwick, Burlington, Ontario

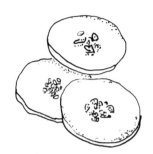

Here is another use for all those zucchinis in the garden. You can vary this recipe with other vegetables—mushrooms, red or green pepper, broccoli. If the handle of the skillet you use is not oven-proof, wrap it in aluminum foil for protection.

2 cups	sliced zucchini	500 mL
1	small onion, minced	1
1 tbsp.	butter or margarine	15 mL
1½ tsp.	olive oil	7 mL
6	eggs, beaten	6
1 tbsp.	chopped parsley	15 mL
1 tsp.	ground fennel	5 mL
½ tsp.	ground rosemary	2 mL
½ tsp.	salt	2 mL
¼ tsp.	freshly ground pepper	1 mL
2 tbsp.	shredded Cheddar cheese	25 mL

In large oven-proof skillet on medium-high heat, cook zucchini and onion in butter and olive oil for about 5 minutes, or until tender.

Combine eggs and seasonings; pour over vegetables. Cook on medium heat without stirring until bottom of mixture has set but top is still soft. Sprinkle cheese on top. Place under preheated broiler about 3 minutes, or until cheese is melted and top is brown.

MENU SUGGESTION
This meatless side dish has a fair amount of fat, so serve it with lower-fat accompaniments. To add a variety of textures, tastes, and colours from each of the four food groups, serve with a fresh fruit combo with orange dressing, Italian Broiled Tomatoes (page 122), corn bread, and café au lait. (Yolanda Jakus, R.P.Dt., London, Ontario)

Preparation: 10 minutes
Cook: about 10 minutes
Makes 6 servings.

Calories per serving: 126
Grams of protein per serving: 7.3
Grams of fat per serving: 9.4
Grams of carbohydrate per serving: 3.1
Grams of fibre per serving: 0.6

LASAGNA ROLL-UPS
Janet Baillie, North York, Ontario

Pasta casseroles can be prepared in stages. Just prepare the filling, the sauce, and the pasta in advance. Then assemble and bake at the last minute. Or complete the dish ahead of time and reheat just before serving.

MENU SUGGESTION
The tofu in this dish combines with noodles and cheese to provide high-quality protein. For a high-fibre vegetarian meal with plenty of vitamins and minerals, serve these roll-ups with a garden fresh salad with low-fat dressing and a multi-grain roll, followed by fresh blueberries with custard sauce. (Mary Sue Waisman, R.D., Calgary, Alberta)

2	large cloves garlic, minced	2
1 tsp.	olive oil	5 mL
2 cups	chopped mushrooms	500 mL
½ cup	diced red pepper	125 mL
1 tsp.	dried thyme	5 mL
1 tsp.	fennel seed	5 mL
¼ tsp.	salt	1 mL
Pinch	black pepper	Pinch
¼ lb.	firm tofu, drained and crumbled	125 g
2 cups	Versatile Tomato Sauce (page 176)	500 mL
6	cooked lasagna noodles	6
1 cup	shredded low-fat mozzarella cheese	250 mL

Preparation: 30 minutes
Cook: about 25 minutes
Makes 6 servings.

Calories per serving: 226
Grams of protein per serving: 12.8
Grams of fat per serving: 6.8
Grams of carbohydrate per serving: 29.9
Grams of fibre per serving: 2.3

In large skillet on medium-high heat, cook garlic in hot oil for about 2 minutes. Add mushrooms, red pepper, and seasonings; cook on high heat, stirring constantly, for about 5 minutes, or until liquid evaporates and vegetables are tender. Add tofu.

Spoon half of tomato sauce into bottom of 8-inch (2 L) square baking pan.

Spread about ⅓ cup (75 mL) mushroom mixture over each cooked noodle. Divide cheese evenly over filling on each noodle. Roll up jelly-roll style. Arrange rolls, seam side down, in baking dish. Spoon remaining tomato sauce over rolls. Cover and bake in 350°F (180°C) oven for 15 minutes; remove cover and bake for about 10 minutes.

LENTIL SPAGHETTI SAUCE
Lise Bélisle, Yamaska, Quebec

Whole wheat, spinach, or plain spaghetti or fettucine, all can be served with Lentil Spaghetti Sauce. Lentils come in two types — brown, which hold their shape and are usually used in salads, and red, which turn soft and mushy when cooked and are the ones we suggest for this recipe.

1	large onion, chopped	1
1	large celery stalk, chopped	1
2	cloves garlic, chopped	2
1 tbsp.	vegetable oil	15 mL
1 cup	dried red lentils, washed	250 mL
2 cups	beef broth or water	500 mL
1	can (5 ½ oz./156 mL) tomato paste	1
¾ cup	water	175 mL
1 tbsp.	chopped fresh parsley	15 mL
½ tsp.	dried oregano	2 mL
½ tsp.	salt	2 mL
Pinch	cayenne pepper	Pinch
	Garnish: grated Parmesan cheese	

MENU SUGGESTION

For an inexpensive meal that provides plenty of complex carbohydrates, protein, and fibre, serve this sauce over your choice of pasta and add colour and texture with a tossed salad with low-cal dressing and Healthy Cheese 'n' Herb Bread (page 199). Round out the meal with Biscuit Baskets with Berry Coulis (page 210). (LeeAnne St. Louis, R.P.Dt., Kitchener, Ontario)

Preparation: 15 minutes
Cook: 45 to 60 minutes
Makes 4 to 6 servings

Calories per serving: 154
Grams of protein per serving: 9.3
Grams of fat per serving: 2.8
Grams of carbohydrate per serving: 25.1
Grams of fibre per serving: 5.1

In large saucepan on medium-high heat, cook onion, celery, and garlic in hot oil for about 5 minutes, or until tender. Add lentils and beef broth; cover and cook on low for about 35 minutes, or until lentils are tender.

Add tomato paste, water, and seasonings; cook covered for about 15 minutes, or until lentils are soft and mushy. Serve over cooked spaghetti; sprinkle with cheese.

WELCOME HOME LENTILS
Christina Mills, Ottawa, Ontario

When Christina Mills sent us her recipe, she commented about lentils, "They cook while I'm at work and welcome me home with a tantalizing aroma at night!" We agree with her. The fragrant aroma of this meatless stew enticed us, too. We enjoyed a bowl with crusty French bread. Cooked rice is another serving possibility. Leftovers freeze well.

Lentils are the seeds of a small shrub plant common in the Mediterranean area. Among the varieties of lentils are red, green, and brown lentils and many types of dhal. Often used as a substitute for meat, lentils are low in fat and relatively inexpensive.

1 tbsp.	olive oil	15 mL
3	medium carrots, sliced	3
6	stalks celery, sliced	6
1	green pepper, diced	1
1	medium Spanish onion, diced	1
3	cloves garlic, minced	3
2 cups	dried lentils	500 mL
1	can (19 oz./540 mL) stewed tomatoes	1
2 cups	vegetable juice cocktail	500 mL
1 tsp.	salt	5 mL
1 tsp.	freshly ground pepper	5 mL
1 tsp.	ground cumin	5 mL
1 tsp.	celery seed	5 mL
1	bay leaf	1
½ tsp.	dried oregano	2 mL
¼ tsp.	cayenne pepper	1 mL

Garnish: plain low-fat yoghurt and shredded low-fat Cheddar cheese

MENU SUGGESTION

Served with crusty sourdough bread, this is a great dish for a cold winter's night. The fat is minimal and the fibre is abundant. For a meal that has plenty of vitamin C (which will optimize the iron absorption in the plant protein in the lentils) serve with confetti coleslaw, followed by Lemon Sherbet (page 224) with orange sections. (Linda Knox, R.P.Dt., Ottawa, Ontario)

In large heavy saucepan on high heat, heat oil. Add carrots, celery, green pepper, onion, and garlic; cook and stir for about 10 minutes, or until vegetables are tender.

Preparation: 30 minutes
Cook: 3 hours or longer
Makes 8 to 10 servings

Calories per serving: 184
Grams of protein per serving: 11.2
Grams of fat per serving: 2.1
Grams of carbohydrate per serving: 32.8
Grams of fibre per serving: 6.5

Transfer to crockpot, heavy stockpot, or oven-proof casserole dish. Add lentils, tomatoes, vegetable juice, and seasonings. Cook, covered, on low for 3 hours or longer, or until lentils are tender or bake, covered, at 250°F (120°C) for 6 to 8 hours. Add extra vegetable juice if mixture becomes too thick.

Serve garnished with yoghurt and Cheddar cheese.

Variation: Cook on the stove using canned lentils; cook just until vegetables are softened and the lentils have absorbed the flavour of the sauce.

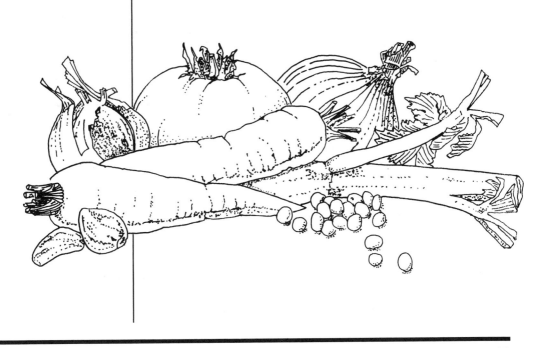

STIR-FRIED VEGETABLES WITH TOFU
Marilyn Peters, Martintown, Ontario

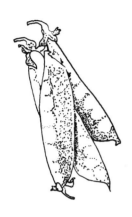

Fresh gingerroot adds an extra zestiness not found in dried ginger and provides a more Oriental authenticity to this recipe. Store tightly wrapped gingerroot in the refrigerator; it will keep for about 7 to 10 days. If you are following a vegetarian diet, use vegetable bouillon instead of chicken bouillon or replace all liquid with tomato juice or vegetable juice cocktail.

Tofu has been a mainstay of the Japanese and Chinese diets. Tofu is made from soy milk, in much the same way that cheese is made from animal milk. It is bland on its own, but takes on the flavour of whatever it is mixed with. It provides protein and some calcium to your recipe. Tofu is best stored in water in a covered container in the refrigerator. Change the water daily to keep tofu fresh for one week.

2 tbsp.	vegetable oil	25 mL
1	large onion, cut into wedges	1
3	medium carrots, sliced diagonally	3
3	celery stalks, sliced diagonally	3
¼	small cabbage, thinly sliced	¼
1 cup	snow peas, trimmed	250 mL
1 cup	sliced mushrooms	250 mL
1 cup	firm tofu, cubed	250 mL
½ cup	chicken broth	125 mL
1 tbsp.	cornstarch	15 mL
1 tsp.	finely chopped gingerroot or	5 mL
½ tsp.	ground ginger	2 mL
¼ tsp.	pepper	1 mL

Preparation: 15 minutes
Cook: 12 minutes
Makes 4 to 6 servings

Calories per serving: 151
Grams of protein per serving: 8.9
Grams of fat per serving: 8.5
Grams of carbohydrate per serving: 12.2
Grams of fibre per serving: 3.6

In wok or large heavy skillet, heat oil over high heat. When oil is very hot, add onion, carrot, and celery; cover and let steam for 5 minutes. Add cabbage, snow peas, mushrooms, and tofu; let steam with cover on for 5 minutes longer.

Mix chicken broth, cornstarch, gingerroot, and pepper; pour over vegetable mixture. Stir-fry for 1 minute, or until sauce thickens. Serve over hot rice.

FALAFEL

Margaret Howard, Toronto, Ontario

Residents of Middle Eastern countries enjoy falafels in much the same way as the hamburger is eaten in North America. Traditionally, falafels are made from cooked chick peas, ground and seasoned, then shaped into balls and deep-fried. Several balls are then placed in pita bread and topped with Tahini Yoghurt Salad. The following adaptation shapes the chick pea mixture into patties and uses much less oil. Seasonings may be increased to suit your taste, and extra bread crumbs will give a drier patty.

MENU SUGGESTION

Chick peas, an excellent source of complex carbohydrates, form the basis of this economical, low-fat, meatless menu. Serve falafels with whole wheat pita pockets, vegetable garnishes, yoghurt, Tabbouleh (page 150), and fresh fruit for additional fibre and texture. (Sharon Parker, R.P.Dt., Willowdale, Ontario)

TAHINI YOGHURT SALAD

Combine plain yoghurt with chopped tomato and cucumber, minced garlic, and parsley; add some tahini paste and freshly ground pepper to taste.

1	can (19 oz./540 mL) chick peas, drained (reserve liquid)	1
2	large cloves garlic	2
1	small onion, cut up	1
½ cup	packed parsley leaves	125 mL
⅓ cup	tahini (sesame seed paste)	75 mL
2 tbsp.	lemon juice	25 mL
1 tbsp.	ground cumin	15 mL
1 tsp.	ground coriander	5 mL
1 tsp.	ground turmeric	5 mL
½ tsp.	salt	2 mL
¼ tsp.	pepper	1 mL
¼ cup	dried bread crumbs	50 mL
1 tbsp.	vegetable oil	15 mL
4	whole wheat pita breads	4
	Garnish: shredded lettuce, chopped tomatoes, diced cucumber, alfalfa sprouts, plain yoghurt	

Preparation: 15 minutes
Cook: 6 minutes
Makes 8 servings

Calories per serving: 253
Grams of protein per serving: 8.7
Grams of fat per serving: 8.4
Grams of carbohydrate per serving: 37.6
Grams of fibre per serving: 3.2

In food processor or blender, process chick peas, 2 tbsp. (25 mL) reserved bean liquid, garlic, onion, parsley, tahini, lemon juice, and seasonings; process until almost smooth. Stir in bread crumbs; shape into 8 patties.

In large non-stick skillet over medium-high heat, heat oil. Add patties, cook for 2 to 3 minutes per side, or until lightly browned. Cut pita breads in half; serve each patty in pocket of one-half pita bread; garnish as desired.

GARBANZOS IN TOMATO SAUCE
Chantal Haddad, St. Laurent, Quebec

Garbanzo beans, also called chick peas, are a protein-filled addition to any recipe. They are commonly available canned or dried. If purchased dried, they will require 2 to 3 hours cooking.

MENU SUGGESTION
This is a welcome low-budget supper choice. For a meal that provides good protein and fibre while supplying only 20 percent of the calories from fat, complement this dish with a spinach salad with low-cal dressing, rye bread, 2 percent milk, and fresh fruit for dessert. (Judy Trépanier, R.P.Dt., Cumberland, Ontario)

1	large onion, cut into thin wedges	1
2	cloves garlic, minced	2
1 tbsp.	olive oil	15 mL
1	can (28 oz./796 mL) garbanzo beans (chick peas), drained	1
1½ cups	canned crushed tomatoes	375 mL
½ tsp.	salt	2 mL
½ tsp.	pepper	2 mL
½ tsp.	dried thyme	2 mL
¼ tsp.	cayenne pepper	1 mL
1	bay leaf	1
	Garnish: chopped fresh parsley	

In large saucepan on medium-high heat, cook onion and garlic in oil for about 5 minutes, or until tender. Add garbanzo beans; cook for 3 to 4 minutes. Add tomatoes and seasonings; cook on low heat for about 25 minutes. Serve garnished with chopped parsley.

Preparation: 10 minutes
Cook: 25 minutes
Makes 4 servings.

Calories per serving: 306
Grams of protein per serving: 11.3
Grams of fat per serving: 5.8
Grams of carbohydrate per serving: 54.4
Grams of fibre per serving: 9.3

SPICY VEGETABLE ENCHILADAS
Lisa Hamilton, Toronto, Ontario

These enchiladas will be softer if cooked in the microwave and crisper if cooked in a conventional oven. Add hot pepper sauce or Mexican salsa to suit your taste.

1	can (14 oz./398 mL) kidney beans, drained	1
1	can (14 oz./398 mL) crushed tomatoes	1
1 cup	firm tofu, cubed	250 mL
½ cup	finely chopped peanuts	125 mL
2 tbsp.	Mexican salsa or hot sauce	25 mL
½ tsp.	chili powder	2 mL
½ tsp.	salt	2 mL
6	large soft corn or flour tortillas	6
1 cup	shredded Monterey Jack or Cheddar cheese	250 mL

In saucepan, combine kidney beans, tomatoes, tofu, peanuts, salsa, and seasonings; heat until hot and bubbling, stirring constantly to prevent sticking.

Spread filling evenly over tortillas; roll tortillas around filling. Place seam side down on a baking sheet; sprinkle with cheese. Bake in 350°F (180°C) oven for about 5 minutes, or microwave on High (100 percent) for about 3 minutes, or until cheese melts.

MENU SUGGESTION

Legumes are a great source of vegetable protein and fibre. The combination of legumes and cereal protein in this Mexican-style recipe ensures a complete protein intake. Skim-milk cheddar cheese may be used to lower the fat content. Serve with cut-up vegetables with chili sauce dip, Spanish rice, and limeade. Round out the meal with pineapple-orange sherbet. (Tracy Hutchings, R.P.Dt., Burlington, Ontario)

Preparation: 15 minutes
Cook: 3 to 5 minutes
Makes 6 large enchiladas

Calories per enchilada: 377
Grams of protein per enchilada: 21.4
Grams of fat per enchilada: 17.3
Grams of carbohydrate per enchilada: 38.1
Grams of fibre per enchilada: 6.4

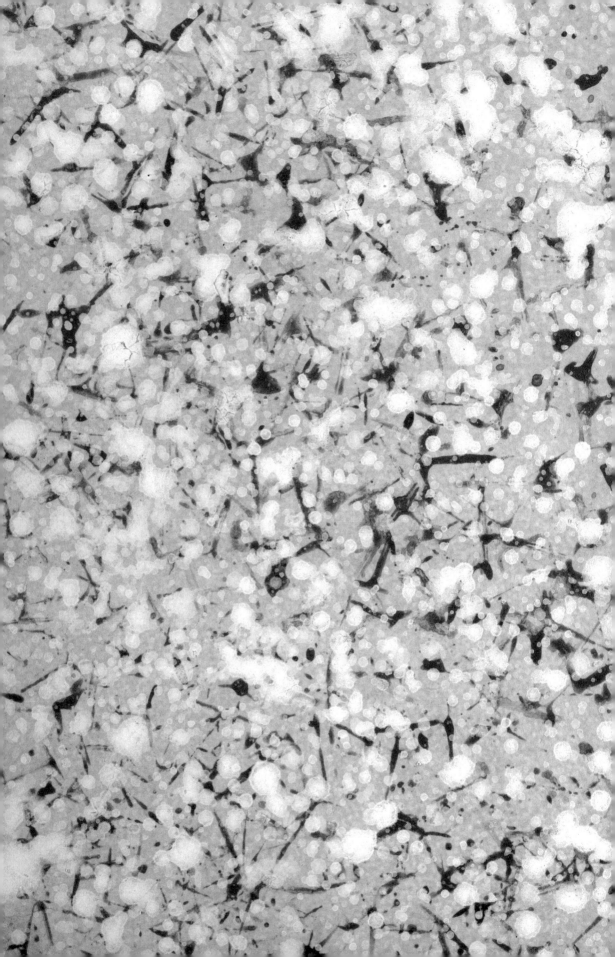

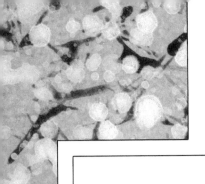

COLOURFUL • DELICIOUS

VEGETABLES

Vegetables were once described as the forgotten guest on the menu. Although nowadays this comment is something of an exaggeration, variety is often still lacking in this particular part of our diet. Yet today, vegetables are becoming more abundant, more available year-round, more numerous, and more varied as well as fresher. Thanks to longer growing seasons and better transportation, they arrive from near and far to benefit our cooking.

COOKING METHODS: Many cooking methods are used in the preparation of vegetables. The microwave is an excellent way to cook vegetables. It preserves flavour, texture, nutritive value, and appearance, as well as being fast and easy. Since microwaved vegetables cook in little or no water, their flavour remains more intense, their texture crisper, and colour more vibrant. Check cooking times for individual vegetables in a microwave cookbook.

Another method, steaming, cooks vegetables as briefly as possible and also helps retain nutrients that leach out during the longer boiling process. For success in steaming, do not overcrowd the vegetables, never let the water touch them, and be sure the container has a tight-fitting cover. The fastest-cooking vegetables are those with the highest water content.

Other methods like sautéing and baking will always be popular, and we have some of these to interest everyone, from Turnip Puff (page 133) and Apple-Stuffed Squash (page 132) to Sautéed Vegetables (page 121).

Vitamins in Vegetables: V for Vitamin; V for Vegetable—they go hand in hand. The vitamin C group includes broccoli, Brussels sprouts, cabbage, cauliflower, chard, green and red peppers, spinach, tomatoes, turnip, and watercress. The vitamin A group includes avocados, broccoli, carrots, chard, pumpkin, spinach, squash, sweet potatoes, and watercress.

Tips on Buying: This subject can be covered in a few brief words. Buy at the peak of freshness. If the vegetable looks fresh—not wilted or withered — it likely has retained its nutrient value. Local produce is your best buy and is generally the best price.

Availability Table of Fresh Canadian-Grown Vegetables

TYPE	SEASON
Asparagus	late April to June
Beans	late June to frost
Beets	late July to April (storage)
Broccoli	early July to late October
Brussels sprouts	August to December
Cabbage	early June to April (storage)
Carrots	late July to May (storage)
Cauliflower	early June to November
Celery	June to November
Sweet corn	mid July to October
Eggplant	August to November
Leeks	August to February (some storage)
Mushrooms	all year
Onions	all year
Parsnips	September to April (storage)
Peas	mid June to August
Peppers	August to October
Potatoes	all year
Rutabaga (Turnip)	August to May (storage)
Spinach	May to October
Summer squash (e.g., zucchini)	mid August to frost (some storage)
Tomatoes	early April to mid December
Winter squash (e.g., Hubbard)	mid August to mid March (some storage)

VITAMIN A CONTENT OF SOME VEGETABLES (½ cup/125 mL)

More than 400 RE*	200-400 RE*	Less than 200 RE*
Carrots, raw or cooked Broccoli, raw Spinach, cooked Sweet potato, cooked Winter squash, cooked	Beet greens, canned Broccoli, cooked	Tomatoes

*Retinol equivalent

VITAMIN C CONTENT OF SOME VEGETABLES (½ cup/125 mL)

More than 40mg	20-40 mg	Less than 20 mg
Broccoli Brussels sprouts Green or red pepper	Cabbage, raw or cooked Cauliflower Potato, baked or boiled Rutabaga, cooked Sweet potato, raw Tomato, fresh or canned Tomato juice	Asparagus Beet greens Potato, mashed Squash, summer or winter Sauerkraut Sweet potato, canned

Health and Welfare Canada

MENU SUGGESTION

Use the sauce in this recipe sparingly, because peanuts and coconut milk are higher in fat. Serve with Salade à la Gout (page 149). Low-fat milk will complement the protein in the peanuts to provide high-quality protein. For dessert, melon sherbet is a refreshing complement to the meal. (Jean Norman, R.Dt., St. John's, Newfoundland)

FRESH VEGETABLE CRÊPES WITH PEANUT SAUCE

Rose Soneff, Penticton, British Columbia

This recipe was inspired by the current interest in Thai cuisine. Like most cooks in Southeast Asia, Thais flavour their dishes with a sauce. This sauce, as well as the crêpes, can be made ahead to allow fast last-minute assembly.

Crêpe batter (use Cottage Cheese-Filled Crêpe recipe, page 101; omit sugar)

PEANUT SAUCE

½ cup	unsweetened coconut milk (available in supermarkets and specialty shops)	125 mL
⅓ cup	crunchy peanut butter	75 mL
2 tbsp.	soy sauce	25 mL
1	clove garlic, minced	1
2 tbsp.	lemon juice	25 mL
1 tsp.	grated lemon rind	5 mL

VEGETABLE FILLING

2 cups	small broccoli florets	500 mL
1½ cups	green beans, chopped	375 mL
1 cup	shredded Savoy cabbage	250 mL
½ cup	carrot strips	125 mL
1 cup	fresh bean sprouts	250 mL
1 tbsp.	chopped fresh coriander	15 mL
	Garnish: fresh coriander, lemon zest or peanut halves	

Preparation: 45 minutes
Cook: about 5 minutes
Makes 8 crêpes or 4 servings of 2 crêpes each

Calories per serving: 356
Grams of protein per serving: 17.7
Grams of fat per serving: 20.4
Grams of carbohydrate per serving: 31.8
Grams of fibre per serving: 7.4

Prepare 8 crêpes; set aside.

To make peanut sauce: In saucepan, combine coconut milk, peanut butter, soy sauce, and garlic. Cook over medium heat, stirring constantly, until smooth and hot. Add lemon juice and rind. Set aside, or keep warm until serving time.

To make vegetable filling: In large pot of boiling water, blanch broccoli, beans, cabbage, and carrot strips for about 2 minutes; rinse under cold water; drain well.

In large bowl, combine bean sprouts, blanched vegetables, and coriander. Place about ⅓ cup (75 mL) vegetable mixture on uncooked side of each crêpe. Roll up crêpes; place seam side down on baking sheet or microwavable dish. Bake, covered, in 350°F (180°C) oven for about 10 minutes, or microwave on High (100 percent) for 2 to 3 minutes.

To serve, top each crêpe with about 1 tbsp. (15 mL) peanut sauce and garnish as desired.

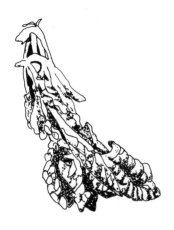

MENU SUGGESTION

Dark green leafy vegetables, such as spinach, are an important source of vitamin A, folate, and iron. This imaginative dish goes well with fish: serve fillets with herbed crumbs, tomato wedges, and oven-baked French fries (leave the skins on the potatoes for extra fibre). Add extra fibre to the meal by serving Sunflower Cookies (page 195) for dessert. (Elaine Power, R.Dt., Port aux Basques, Newfoundland)

Preparation: 10 minutes
Cook: 4 to 5 minutes
Makes 4 to 5 servings

Calories per serving: 50
Grams of protein per serving: 1.8
Grams of fat per serving: 2.4
Grams of carbohydrate per serving: 6.7
Grams of fibre per serving: 1.5

SPINACH FANCY
Martine Lortie, Ste-Foy, Quebec

No one will have to tell you to eat your spinach any more! You will be more than willing to prepare and enjoy this version.

1	bag (10 oz./284 g) fresh spinach	1
3 tbsp.	raisins	45 mL
Pinch	dried mint	Pinch
Pinch	ground fennel	Pinch
Pinch	dried oregano	Pinch
1 tbsp.	butter or margarine	15 mL
2 tbsp.	water	25 mL
1 tsp.	lemon juice	5 mL
½ tsp.	salt	2 mL
Pinch	pepper	Pinch
	Garnish: lemon slices	

Wash spinach and dry thoroughly; remove stems and chop.

In large skillet on medium heat, cook raisins, mint, fennel, and oregano in butter. Add spinach and water; cover and steam for 2 to 3 minutes, or until wilted. Drain liquid. Sprinkle with lemon juice, salt, and pepper; toss well. Serve with lemon slices.

SAUTÉED VEGETABLES
Jeanette Snowden, Milton, Ontario

What is unusual in this vegetable sauté is the addition of chopped beets, which provide an attractive rosy red colour to the dish. You may want to serve this colourful mix of vegetables over white rice.

¼ cup	sliced onion	50 mL
1 tbsp.	olive oil	15 mL
1 cup	broccoli florets	250 mL
1 cup	cauliflower florets	250 mL
1 cup	cubed zucchini	250 mL
½ cup	chopped raw beets	125 mL
1 cup	chicken broth	250 mL
1 cup	chopped Swiss chard or spinach (optional)	250 mL
1 cup	chopped tomatoes	250 mL
2 tbsp.	water	25 mL
2 tsp.	cornstarch	10 mL
	Salt and pepper to taste	

In large skillet on medium-high heat, cook onion in hot oil for about 5 minutes. Add broccoli, cauliflower, zucchini, beets, and chicken broth. Cook, covered, for about 3 minutes, or until crisp-tender.

Stir in chard (if using) and tomatoes. Mix water, cornstarch, and seasonings; stir into vegetable mixture. Cook for about 2 minutes, or until thickened.

Fresh beets are delicious steamed or cold in salads. There's an easy way to cook them to get their best flavour and nutrition. Cut the green tops from beets, leaving at least one inch attached. Don't remove the root end. This prevents the beet colour and vitamins from being lost in the cooking water. Once the beets are cooked, rinse under cold water and slide off the beet skins. Rubber gloves are good to use for this job.

MENU SUGGESTION

Surround this vegetable combo with braised chicken wings (or breasts, which would be lower in fat) and steamed rice, followed by date pudding with orange sauce and voilà . . . an appetizing meal providing many vitamins and minerals, especially potassium, niacin, and vitamin C. (Elizabeth Farrell, P.Dt., Saint John, New Brunswick)

Preparation: 20 minutes
Cook: 15 minutes
Makes 6 servings

Calories per serving: 53
Grams of protein per serving: 2.5
Grams of fat per serving: 2.6
Grams of carbohydrate per serving: 6.1
Grams of fibre per serving: 2.0

LIGHTLY GLAZED STIR-FRIED VEGETABLES

Doris Pennell, Corner Brook, Newfoundland

Not all stir-fry recipes are created equal. Here's one without soy sauce. Chicken broth replaces much of the oil used in a traditional stir-fry, thus helping this dish live up to the name "lightly glazed."

Try pouring low-cal bottled dressings over hot vegetables (like broccoli and cauliflower) instead of butter and margarine.

2 tbsp.	peanut oil	25 mL
2 cups	cauliflower florets	500 mL
2 cups	broccoli florets	500 mL
1 cup	diagonally sliced carrot	250 mL
1 cup	diagonally sliced celery	250 mL
3	green onions, sliced	3
1	small red pepper, thinly sliced	1
1	small green pepper, thinly sliced	1
2	chicken bouillon cubes	2
1 cup	boiling water	250 mL
2 tsp.	garlic powder	10 mL
1 tsp.	onion powder	5 mL
¼ tsp.	white pepper	1 mL
1 tbsp.	cornstarch	15 mL
2 tbsp.	water	25 mL

MENU SUGGESTION

This flavourful vegetable dish adds colour and crunch to any menu. Serve with fish fillets with basil and lemon and parsley potatoes for a meal that provides a generous amount of fibre and vitamins with minimal fat. For a refreshing finish to the meal, serve strawberry mousse. (Elaine Power, R.Dt., Port aux Basques, Newfoundland)

Heat wok until very hot. (To test if hot enough, a drop of water in the wok should sizzle and evaporate instantly.) Add oil; heat until very hot. Add cauliflower, broccoli, carrot, celery, and green onions; stir-fry for 2 to 3 minutes. Add red and green pepper; stir-fry for 2 minutes.

Dissolve chicken bouillon in boiling water; stir in seasonings and add to wok. Cover and steam for about 2 minutes, or until vegetables are crisp-tender.

Photos: Deluxe Peas, page 125 (facing page); Cheesy Broccoli and Potato Casserole, page 128 (overleaf)

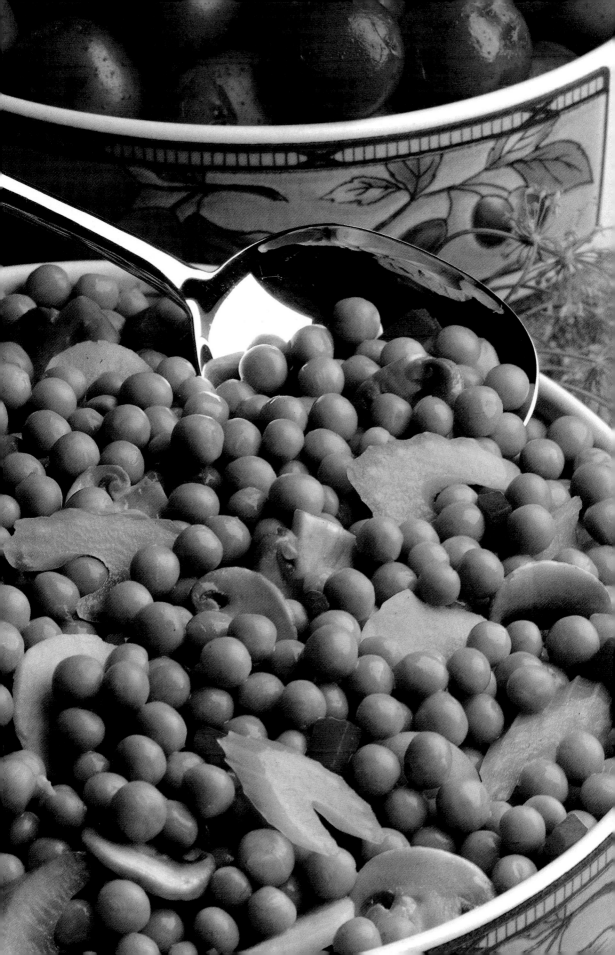

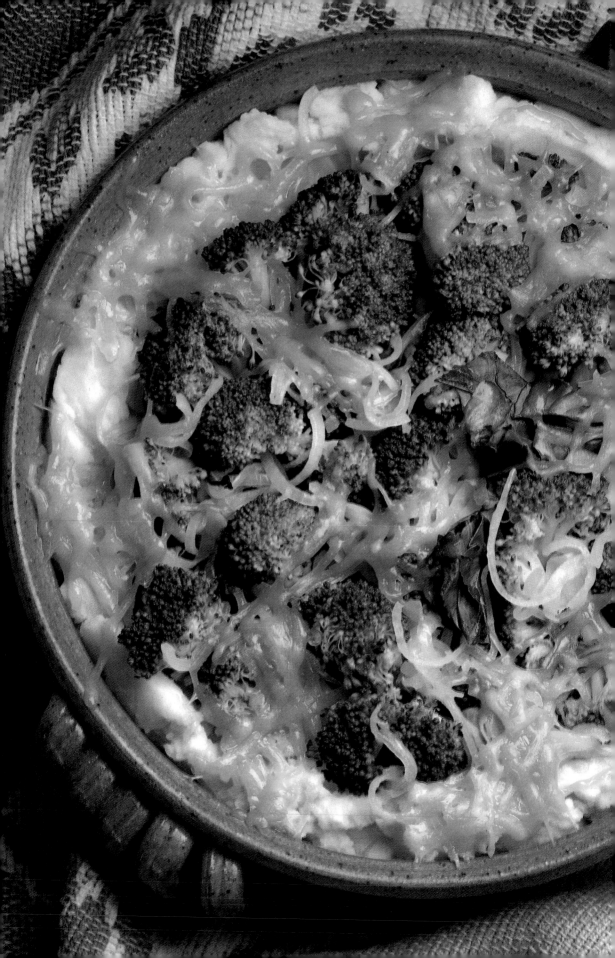

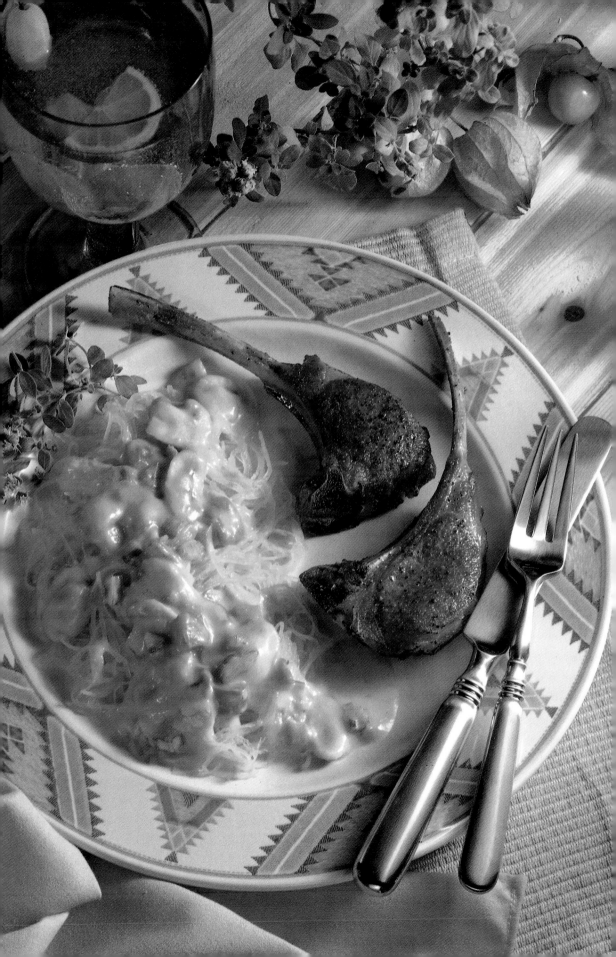

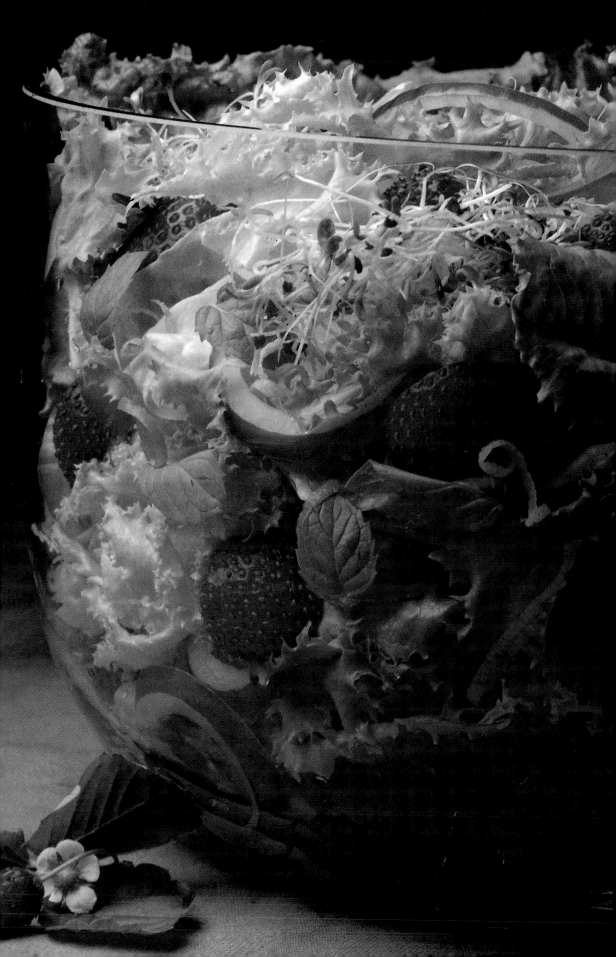

Preparation: 25 minutes
Cook: 10 minutes
Makes 6 servings

Calories per serving: 91
Grams of protein per serving: 3.3
Grams of fat per serving: 4.7
Grams of carbohydrate per serving: 11.1
Grams of fibre per serving: 3.5

Combine 2 tbsp. (25 mL) water with cornstarch. Slowly stir into vegetables; turn vegetables frequently to coat with sauce.

Variation: Mary Ellen Langlois of Sudbury, Ontario, sent us her Colourful Vegetable Stir-Fry recipe. Her recipe suggests using yellow cooking onions, bean sprouts, miniature corn cobs, and snow peas with some of the same vegetables used above.

Pansy Jacobs from St. Anthony, Newfoundland, uses celery, cabbage, and mushrooms, as well as other vegetables, in her Stir-Fry Vegetable recipe.

What are cruciferous vegetables? These vegetables come from the Cruciferae (mustard) family. The name comes from the vegetables' characteristic four-petaled, cross-shaped flower. Crucifers include broccoli, brussels sprouts, cabbage, cauliflower, kohlrabi, kale, and rutabaga. Cook these vegetables uncovered for a few minutes then cover. Their flavour and colour will be better without sacrificing too much nutrient value.

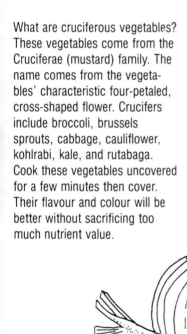

Photos: Spaghetti Squash with Mushrooms, page 130 (overleaf); Variety Greens with Fresh Strawberries, page 139 (facing page)

121

The debate rages on — is a tomato a fruit or a vegetable? A United States Supreme Court decision in 1893 legally made the tomato a vegetable. But whatever you think, treat your tomatoes carefully. Store underripe tomatoes unwashed, at room temperature away from sunlight, until slightly soft. Room temperature tomatoes will have more flavour than cold ones.

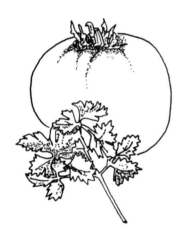

ITALIAN BROILED TOMATOES
Helen Haresign, Toronto, Ontario

Serve this often during tomato season to accompany broiled or barbecued meat.

2	large tomatoes	2
Dash	garlic powder	Dash
1 tbsp.	chopped parsley	15 mL
1 tsp.	dried basil	5 mL
½ tsp.	dried oregano	2 mL
	Freshly ground pepper	
2 tbsp.	bread crumbs	25 mL

Cut tomatoes in half crosswise. Place, cut side up, on rack in shallow baking pan. Sprinkle lightly with garlic powder. Combine parsley, seasonings, and bread crumbs. Divide mixture over surface of tomato halves.

Place pan about 6 inches (15 cm) below broiler. Broil for 3 to 4 minutes until tomatoes are heated through, or cook on the barbecue along with the meat.

Preparation: 10 minutes
Broil: 4 minutes
Makes 4 servings

Calories per serving: 30
Grams of protein per serving: 1.6
Grams of fat per serving: 1.0
Grams of carbohydrate per serving: 4.4
Grams of fibre per serving: 1.2

Red cabbage adds attractive colour to salads but tends to change colour when cooked. The German custom of cooking red cabbage with apples and a small amount of vinegar is not just for added flavour. The addition of an acidic food helps the cabbage keep its nice red colour. Cutting the red cabbage with a stainless steel knife also keeps the red colour from changing.

Preparation: 15 minutes
Cook: 1 hour
Makes 6 servings

Calories per serving: 185
Grams of protein per serving: 1.5
Grams of fat per serving: 7.9
Grams of carbohydrate per serving: 30.2
Grams of fibre per serving: 3.8

SWEET AND SOUR RED CABBAGE
Cathy Collard, Sherwood, Prince Edward Island

Sweet-sour red cabbage is a very popular vegetable in Germany, Russia, and Poland. Since red cabbage requires longer cooking time than green, it is generally shredded or sliced to speed up cooking.

½ cup	chopped onion	125 mL
¼ cup	butter or margarine	50 mL
8 cups	coarsely sliced red cabbage (about 1 medium)	2 L
4	whole cloves	4
1 cup	red wine	250 mL
2	bay leaves	2
4	medium apples, peeled and sliced	4
⅓ cup	brown sugar	75 mL
2 tbsp.	vinegar	25 mL

In large saucepan on medium-high heat, cook onion in butter until slightly soft. Add cabbage, cloves, wine, and bay leaves; cook, covered, about 6 minutes, or until limp.

In large casserole or Dutch oven, layer one-third cabbage mixture and one-third apple slices; sprinkle with some sugar. Repeat layers twice more. Pour vinegar on top. Bake in 325°F (160°C) oven for about 1 hour, or until tender, stirring occasionally; remove bay leaves and cloves before serving.

BRAISED CABBAGE
Alma R. Price, Toronto, Ontario

Lightly cooked green cabbage accepts a variety of interesting seasonings, like the back bacon in this recipe, which is lower in fat than side bacon.

3	slices back bacon, diced	3
1	small onion, sliced	1
¼ cup	finely diced carrot	50 mL
4 cups	shredded cabbage	1 L
1	bay leaf	1
Pinch	dried thyme	Pinch
¼ cup	chicken broth	50 mL
	Freshly ground pepper to taste	

In large skillet on low heat, cook bacon and onion for about 5 minutes, stirring frequently. Add carrot; cover and cook for 1 minute. Stir in cabbage, bay leaf, thyme, and chicken broth. Cook, covered, on low heat for about 10 minutes, or until crisp-tender; stir occasionally. Season to taste with freshly ground pepper. Remove bay leaf before serving.

Preparation: 10 minutes
Cook: 15 minutes
Makes 4 servings

Calories per serving: 71
Grams of protein per serving: 3.5
Grams of fat per serving: 3.2
Grams of carbohydrate per serving: 8.4
Grams of fibre per serving: 3.2

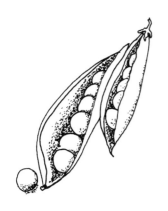

DELUXE PEAS
Donna E. Cronmiller, Winnipeg, Manitoba

As Donna Cronmiller says, Deluxe Peas turns a family favourite into company fare.

1 tbsp.	butter or margarine	15 mL
1 tsp.	chicken bouillon powder	5 mL
2 tbsp.	water	25 mL
1½ cups	sliced mushrooms	375 mL
1 cup	diagonally sliced celery	250 mL
½ tsp.	dried dill weed	2 mL
¼ tsp.	curry powder	1 mL
1	package (350 g) frozen peas	1
¾ cup	sliced water chestnuts	175 mL
2 tbsp.	chopped pimento or red pepper (optional)	25 mL

In large skillet on medium heat, melt butter; stir in chicken bouillon powder, water, mushrooms, celery, and seasonings; cook for about 6 minutes, or until vegetables are almost tender. Stir in peas; cook, covered, for 2 minutes. Add water chestnuts and pimento (if using). Cook for about 1 minute, or until heated through; stir occasionally.

MENU SUGGESTION
Serve with chilled cucumber soup, lemon-herbed barbecued chicken breasts, and wild rice for a meal that provides plenty of dietary fibre. Complete the meal with Strawberry Sorbet (page 223) with fresh strawberries. (Yolanda Jakus, R.P.Dt., London, Ontario)

Preparation: 15 minutes
Cook: about 10 minutes
Makes 6 servings

Calories per serving: 83
Grams of protein per serving: 3.5
Grams of fat per serving: 2.2
Grams of carbohydrate per serving: 12.9
Grams of fibre per serving: 3.0

CARROT ROLLS

Laura M. Hawthorn, Bracebridge, Ontario

Here's a way to dress-up an everyday vegetable. This recipe makes a large number of rolls, but they freeze very well. Mashed potatoes would also work equally well.

MENU SUGGESTION

This is a simple and appealing way to serve this vitamin-A-rich vegetable, but the dish contains more than 6 grams of fat per serving, so keep the rest of the meal lower in fat. Combine with haddock fillets in lemon juice, garnished with toasted almonds, broccoli, and oven-roasted potatoes for a well-balanced meal providing plenty of protein, fibre, and vitamins. Fresh fruit cup is a good choice for dessert. (Lynn Burdock, R.Dt., Halifax, Nova Scotia)

8 cups	sliced carrots	2 L
3 cups	soft bread crumbs	750 mL
2 cups	shredded Cheddar cheese	500 mL
	Salt, pepper, and nutmeg to taste	
2	egg whites	2
1 cup	crushed corn flakes (about 3 cups/ 750 mL corn flakes)	250 mL
	Garnish: parsley sprigs	

Steam carrots for about 10 minutes, or until soft. Drain and mash well. Add bread crumbs, cheese, and seasonings.

Beat egg whites until stiff; fold into carrot mixture. Shape mixture into twenty-four 2-inch (5-cm) long rolls. Roll in crushed corn flakes. Place on non-stick or lightly greased baking sheet. Bake in 350°F (180°C) oven for about 20 minutes, or until brown. Serve garnished with parsley.

Preparation: 30 minutes
Cook: 20 minutes
Makes 24 rolls or 12 servings

Calories per serving: 159
Grams of protein per serving: 7.3
Grams of fat per serving: 6.7
Grams of carbohydrate per serving: 17.9
Grams of fibre per serving: 2.5

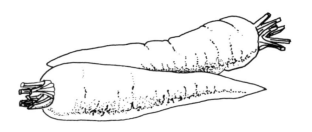

Consumers often ask what causes a potato to go green. Greening is an undesirable but normal colour change when a potato is exposed to light. The greenish colour is a substance called solanine. Don't eat green potatoes. Besides giving a bitter flavour, eating large quantities of them can make you sick. To prevent greening, keep your potatoes in the dark.

MENU SUGGESTION

This calcium-rich pie is colourful, economical, and easy to prepare. The higher amount of fat could be reduced by substituting a low-fat cheese. For a satisfying meal that provides generous amounts of protein, iron, and vitamin C, serve with hearty Beef Barley Soup (page 71), asparagus tips with white sauce, and tomato wedges, followed by Peachy Upside-Down Cake (page 208). (Elizabeth Farrell, P.Dt., Saint John, New Brunswick)

Preparation: 20 minutes
Cook: 40 minutes
Makes 6 servings

Calories per serving: 233
Grams of protein per serving: 10.7
Grams of fat per serving: 10.9
Grams of carbohydrate per serving: 23.8
Grams of fibre per serving: 2.6

RED AND WHITE POTATO DELIGHT PIE
Rose Telfer, Hamilton, Ontario

We're used to eating vegetables individually, but in combination vegetables offer a wide range of flavours and colours. Serve this dish for a buffet dinner party or at a barbecue.

4	slices side bacon, diced	4
2	large onions, finely chopped	2
½	green pepper, finely chopped	½
1	stalk celery, finely chopped	1
3	large potatoes, peeled, coarsely chopped	3
2	tomatoes, coarsely chopped	2
1 cup	shredded old Cheddar cheese	250 mL
2	eggs, separated	2
1 tbsp.	2 percent milk	15 mL
¼ tsp.	salt	1 mL
¼ tsp.	pepper	1 mL

In skillet, cook bacon until almost crisp; remove and drain on paper towel. Add onion, green pepper, and celery to skillet; cook on medium-high for about 5 minutes; drain fat.

Partially cook potatoes in boiling water for 10 minutes; drain well. In non-stick or lightly greased 8-inch (2 L) square baking dish, layer half potatoes, tomatoes, bacon and onion mixture, and cheese; repeat layers.

Whisk together egg yolks and milk. Beat egg whites, salt, and pepper until foamy. Fold egg whites into egg-yolk mixture; pour over vegetables. Bake in 350°F (180°C) oven for about 40 minutes, or until mixture has set.

CHEESY BROCCOLI AND POTATO CASSEROLE

Mary Jo Ennett, Wallaceburg, Ontario

These two widely available vegetables, when combined, provide a comforting and homey casserole.

MENU SUGGESTION

For a wonderful contrast with this creamy fibre-rich casserole, serve chicken breasts with a crunchy sesame-seed coating, cherry tomatoes, and rye bread. Follow with raspberries and blueberries for a meal that keeps calories and fat to a minimum and is easy to prepare. (Christine Williams, R.P.Dt., Belleville, Ontario)

6	medium potatoes, cubed	6
¼ cup	2 percent milk	50 mL
1 tsp.	butter or margarine	5 mL
½ tsp.	white pepper	2 mL
½ tsp.	dried parsley	2 mL
2 cups	broccoli florets	500 mL
1	small onion, sliced	1
1 cup	shredded old Cheddar cheese	250 mL

In large saucepan, cook potatoes in boiling water until tender; drain well. Mash potatoes with milk, butter and seasonings.

Meanwhile, steam broccoli and onion until barely tender, or microwave on High (100 percent) for 5 to 8 minutes.

In lightly greased 8-cup (2 L) casserole, spread potato mixture; top with broccoli, onion, and cheese. Bake, covered, in 350°F (180°C) oven for 10 minutes; remove cover, bake 5 minutes longer, or until cheese is melted. Or microwave, covered, on High (100 percent) for about 8 minutes.

Preparation: 20 minutes
Cook: 15 minutes
Makes 6 servings

Calories per serving: 223
Grams of protein per serving: 9.2
Grams of fat per serving: 7.4
Grams of carbohydrate per serving: 31.8
Grams of fibre per serving: 3.8

PARSNIP SCALLOP
Irene Ferguson, Winnipeg, Manitoba

This scallop of parsnips and carrots is equally as good using only parsnips. The addition of the small amount of sugar heightens the natural sweetness of both parsnips and carrots.

1 ½ lb.	parsnips, cut into coins, or combination of sliced parsnips and carrots	750 g
¼ cup	chopped onion	50 mL
3 tbsp.	butter or margarine	45 mL
3 tbsp.	all-purpose flour	45 mL
1 tsp.	granulated sugar	5 mL
½ tsp.	dried basil	2 mL
½ tsp.	salt	2 mL
Dash	pepper	Dash
2 cups	tomato juice	500 mL
½ cup	dried bread crumbs	125 mL
1 tbsp.	melted butter or margarine	15 mL

Cook parsnips in boiling water for 5 to 10 minutes or just until tender (do not overcook as they fall apart and become mushy); drain well.

In skillet on medium-high heat, cook onion in butter for about 5 minutes. Blend in flour, sugar, and seasonings. Gradually add tomato juice; cook, stirring constantly, for about 5 minutes, or until thickened.

Combine parsnips and tomato sauce in lightly greased casserole. Mix bread crumbs and melted butter; sprinkle over parsnips. Bake in 375°F (190°C) oven for 15 minutes, or until brown.

MENU SUGGESTION
The creamy sauce makes this a higher-fat vegetable choice. Balance it with baked whitefish for protein and brown rice and green peas for a generous fibre intake. Finish the meal with kiwi and orange slices topped with low-fat yoghurt. (Heather More, R.D., Winnipeg, Manitoba)

Preparation: 15 minutes
Cook: 15 minutes
Makes 6 servings

Calories per serving: 225
Grams of protein per serving: 3.7
Grams of fat per serving: 8.2
Grams of carbohydrate per serving: 36.6
Grams of fibre per serving: 4.7

Spaghetti squash is easily recognized by its oblong shape and pale to bright yellow skin. It bakes and microwaves quite easily. When cooked, the flesh separates into spaghetti-like strands. This squash is perfect to mix with all kinds of sauces. Try it in place of pasta with your favourite sauce.

MENU SUGGESTION

The sauce in this recipe is a significant source of fat, so serve it sparingly. This dish goes well with Blond Sangria (page 238), curried lamb chops, Dilly Bread (page 186), and mint gelatine dessert with low-fat yoghurt. (Elizabeth Farrell, P.Dt., Saint John, New Brunswick)

Spaghetti squash is most readily available from August through to November.

SPAGHETTI SQUASH WITH MUSHROOMS
Marlyn Ambrose-Chase, Moose Jaw, Saskatchewan

Spaghetti squash, once cooked, looks just like golden strands of spaghetti, yet tastes like squash. To keep the strands intact, be sure to cut squash in half lengthwise. Since spaghetti squash acts like both pasta and vegetable, you can serve it with your favourite spaghetti sauce, or try Lentil Spaghetti Sauce (page 107).

1	spaghetti squash (about 3½ lb./1.5 kg)	1
2 tbsp.	butter or margarine	25 mL
2 cups	sliced mushrooms	500 mL
2 cups	chopped tomatoes (4 small)	500 mL
1	green onion, sliced	1
1	small stalk celery, chopped	1
2 tbsp.	all-purpose flour	25 mL
1 cup	2 percent milk	250 mL
½ cup	shredded Cheddar cheese	125 mL
1 tsp.	dried oregano	5 mL
½ tsp.	garlic powder	2 mL
½ tsp.	salt	2 mL
¼ tsp.	freshly ground pepper	1 mL
	Garnish: grated Parmesan cheese	

Microwave instructions: Pierce whole squash with a fork in several places; place on double thickness of paper towel and microwave on High (100 percent) for 10 minutes, turning over halfway through. Slice squash in half lengthwise; remove seeds. Cover squash halves with vented plastic wrap and cook on High for 10 to 15 minutes, or until tender; rotate squash twice. Let stand for 5 minutes. With a fork, remove spaghetti-like strands of squash; place in bowl, season to taste. Cover and keep warm.

To make sauce: In 4-cup (1 L) microwavable casserole, melt butter on High (100 percent) for 30 seconds. Stir in mushrooms, onion, celery, and tomatoes. Microwave, uncovered, on High (100 percent) for about 3 minutes, or until vegetables are tender. Stir in flour; gradually add milk, microwave on High for 4 minutes, or until mixture comes to a boil and thickens; stir twice. Add Cheddar cheese and seasonings; stir until cheese is melted.

Pour mushroom sauce over spaghetti squash; sprinkle with Parmesan cheese and serve.

Preparation: 15 minutes
Cook: about 35 minutes
Makes 6 servings

Calories per serving: 163
Grams of protein per serving: 6.1
Grams of fat per serving: 8.2
Grams of carbohydrate per serving: 18.0
Grams of fibre per serving: 3.6

Conventional oven directions: Cut squash in half lengthwise. Bake in 350°F (180°C) oven for 25 to 30 minutes, cut side down, on a baking sheet or boil, covered, cut side down, in 2 inches (5 cm) of water for about 20 minutes.

To make sauce: In skillet on medium-high heat, cook mushrooms, onion, celery, and tomatoes in butter for about 5 minutes, or until tender. Stir in flour; gradually add milk. Cook, stirring constantly, until thickened. Stir in Cheddar cheese and seasonings until cheese is melted.

Pour sauce over squash; sprinkle with Parmesan cheese and serve.

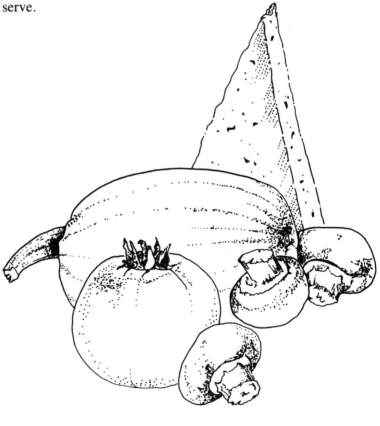

Have you ever wrestled with a large hard-shelled squash you want to cut in pieces? Here's an easy method to cut it open. First split off the stem. With a large, sharp knife, pierce the skin of the squash where you want to cut it. Insert your knife slightly into the squash and tap it several times with a hammer or meat mallet. The squash should split on its own.

MENU SUGGESTION

Prepare this highly flavoured side dish as an accompaniment to roast pork. The main source of fat in the recipe is the nuts. All you need to complete the meal is Spinach Salad with Creamy Garlic Dressing (page 136) and a dish of brown rice for a dinner that's high in fibre, thiamin, and iron. Peach melba completes the meal and contributes some calcium. (Yolanda Jakus, R.P.Dt., London, Ontario)

Preparation: 10 minutes
Cook: about 50 minutes
Makes 4 servings

Calories per serving: 323
Grams of protein per serving: 3.6
Grams of fat per serving: 7.7
Grams of carbohydrate per serving: 67.7
Grams of fibre per serving: 6.1

APPLE-STUFFED SQUASH
Irene Mofina, Shannonville, Ontario

Squash, a favourite homegrown fall vegetable, makes a wonderful container for rice, meats, or fruit. Conserve energy by baking potatoes and meat at the same time.

2	acorn squash	2
2 cups	unsweetened apple sauce	500 mL
½ cup	raisins	125 mL
¼ cup	honey or molasses	50 mL
¼ cup	chopped walnuts	50 mL
1 tbsp.	butter or margarine	15 mL
1 tbsp.	grated lemon rind	15 mL
2 tsp.	lemon juice	10 mL
¼ tsp.	ground cinnamon	1 mL

Cut squash in half; remove seeds. Combine apple sauce, raisins, honey, and walnuts. Fill squash with mixture; dot each squash with butter. Sprinkle with lemon rind, juice, and cinnamon.

Place filled squash in shallow baking pan; pour hot water to ¼-inch (1 cm) depth. Bake, covered, in 375°F (190°C) oven for 30 minutes; uncover dish, bake another 20 minutes, or until squash is tender.

TURNIP PUFF
Nadia Martin, Eden Mills, Ontario

*Cooked turnip or squash are both excellent in this mild, delicate
vegetable casserole.*

½ cup	chopped onion	125 mL
1 tbsp.	melted butter or margarine, divided	15 mL
3 cups	cooked, mashed turnip	750 mL
2	eggs, separated	2
¼ cup	skim milk	50 mL
3 tbsp.	all-purpose flour	45 mL
1 tbsp.	baking powder	15 mL
½ tsp.	salt	2 mL
¼ tsp.	ground nutmeg	1 mL
Dash	freshly ground pepper	Dash
½ cup	whole wheat bread crumbs	125 mL

Cook onion in non-stick skillet in 1 tsp. (5 mL) butter
until tender. Add to mashed turnip.

Beat egg whites until stiff; set aside. Beat egg yolks with
milk; stir in flour, baking powder, and seasonings. Stir
egg-yolk mixture into mashed turnip. Fold in beaten egg
whites.

Turn into lightly greased 6-cup (1.5 L) baking dish.
Combine bread crumbs and remaining melted butter.
Sprinkle over turnip. Bake in 375°F (190°C) oven for
about 30 minutes.

Preparation: 20 minutes
Cook: about 30 minutes
Makes 6 servings

Calories per serving: 119
Grams of protein per serving:
4.7
Grams of fat per serving: 4.3
Grams of carbohydrate per
serving: 16.6
Grams of fibre per serving: 2.9

SALADS

A few years back, the produce manager in a supermarket was overheard to say that salads and salad dressings sell primarily in the summer. Not so now—today's consumer enjoys salads year-round.

Once upon a time, three types of lettuce were available: iceberg, romaine, and Boston. Today, produce sections offer an exciting variety of ingredients, from fancy lettuces, like bibb, radicchio, watercress, and red leaf lettuce, to snow peas, Belgian endive, and fresh herbs. The proverbial "tossed greens" salad is almost a thing of the past. You can also spark a salad with citrus fruits, pears, apples, kiwi fruit, and even strawberries.

Following are a few of the new salad ingredients:

Radicchio: a relatively new delicacy from Italy, radicchio is a member of the chicory family. One or two leaves used as a garnish or torn up with other greens will dramatically enhance a simple salad.

Arugula: small, tender, and pungent with dark green leaves, arugula adds a spicy taste to sweet or bitter greens.

Belgian endive: the pale green, almost white spear-like leaves of Belgian endive form a small, compact head that is crisp-textured and juicy; use for arranged salads or as dippers.

Select ingredients according to the season, always buying fresh ingredients in spring and summer. In winter, the Winter Vegetable Salad (page 144) and Carrot and Orange Salad with Yoghurt (page 138) are less expensive to prepare than lettuce salads. And substituting spinach for the traditional tossed greens can be cost effective.

Eye appeal is important. Creative arrangement of foods should not be left just to magazine and cookbook food stylists. You too can be creative in assembling salads with eye and appetite appeal. On a lettuce leaf, place orange segments and snow pea pods, drizzle with the yogurt dressing used for Golden Treasure Salad (page 143), sprinkle with sunflower seeds for added crunch. The eye appeal—to say nothing of the nutritive value—of this salad is superb.

WINDOWSILL GARDENING

Fresh herbs are hot news these days. Use them garden-fresh in summer, and keep potfuls on sunny windowsills in winter.

Which to choose? Oregano, cilantro, bay, lemon thyme, rosemary, sweet marjoram, and tarragon can all be grown successfully. Parsley, dill, chives, and basil are now becoming so common it's better not to waste time or space on them.

Invest in good soil, terra cotta pots with saucers (because they absorb and release moisture) and a good plant food. Do not overwater; most herbs are killed this way. South light is best, although they will grow on eastern or western exposures.

To store, rinse herbs in cool water. Pick over the best leaves, discard stems. Dry well; store in refrigerator for up to 1 week in a sealed plastic bag with paper towels to absorb moisture.

To convert recipes from fresh to dried herbs, use 1 tbsp. (15 mL) of a fresh herb to equal 1 tsp. (5 mL) dried.

For garnishes, try herbs other than parsley. Mint, basil or tarragon leaves, and feathery dill are appropriate, as are pale green celery leaves and carrot tops.

HOW TO MAKE A SALAD A MEAL

Main-course salads are becoming a big feature in today's cooking. Any pasta, rice, or potato salad with the addition of protein — salmon, tuna, ham, chicken, cold roast beef or pork, hard-cooked eggs, or cheese — can become a main-course meal. Add to this a green vegetable salad, sliced tomatoes or marinated cucumbers, and a sprinkle of fresh herbs, and you have a satisfying entrée. Round out the meal with a hearty bread and a glass of milk.

HERB VINEGARS

Herb vinegars can add exciting flavours to salads and help reduce the amount of oil needed.

To make your own herb vinegar, pick herbs before they flower; bruise the leaves slightly to help release flavour. Place herbs in clean, sterilized jars. Cover with your choice of vinegar (red, white, or rice). Be sure to purchase good, not cheap vinegars. The best ratio is ⅔ cup (150 mL) packed fresh herbs to 1 cup (250 mL) vinegar.

Steep for about 2 weeks in a warm, dark place; shake occasionally. Strain and bottle. For a nice touch, add a fresh sprig of the herb used in each bottle. Cork and store in a cool place.

WHAT'S SPECIAL ABOUT SPECIALTY OILS?

It may seem odd to be discussing oils in a cookbook with an emphasis on low fat; however, in small quantities, oils can provide distinctive flavours to food. Take olive oil, for example. If used instead of vegetable oil in a stir-fry, a more robust flavour will result.

Some of the more sophisticated oils — walnut, sesame, peanut — also add unique flavours to food. If these specialty oils are used in salad dressings, a smaller amount is needed, since they enhance and lend distinction to the dressing. Be aware: this distinction carries a price tag. These oils are more expensive. And they are not recommended in highly seasoned recipes, or where their special flavours will be hidden.

SPINACH SALAD WITH CREAMY GARLIC DRESSING
Gail P. Foster, St. Lazare, Quebec

Homemade whole wheat croutons and yoghurt dressing create a new and light version of this popular salad.

DRESSING

½ cup	low-fat plain yoghurt	125 mL
¼ cup	chopped fresh parsley	50 mL
2 tbsp.	light mayonnaise	25 mL
1	large clove garlic, minced	1
Pinch	salt, pepper	Pinch

1	slice whole wheat bread	1
10 cups	spinach leaves	2.5 L
1½ cups	sliced mushrooms	375 mL
¼ cup	alfalfa sprouts	50 mL
2 tbsp.	grated Parmesan cheese	25 mL

Cut bread into cubes; toast in 350°F (180°C) oven for 5 minutes, or until crisp and brown.

Tear spinach into bite-size pieces. In large salad bowl, combine toasted bread cubes, spinach, mushrooms, alfalfa sprouts, and Parmesan cheese.

Combine yoghurt, parsley, mayonnaise, garlic, salt, and pepper. Pour dressing over vegetables; toss until well coated.

Variation: Add ½ cup (125 mL) of one of the following: chopped apple, mandarin orange, red or green peppers, tomatoes, or red onion.

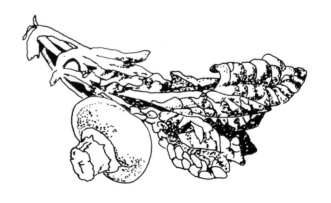

MENU SUGGESTION

This salad is low in calories and fat but still has a rich garlic flavour. Serve with roast pork tenderloin with savoury seasoning, oven roasted potatoes with parsley, and Steamed Brown Bread (page 203) for a variety packed nutritional feast. Finish the meal with refreshing multi-melon sorbet with mint. (Barbara Winder, R.P.Dt., Hamilton, Ontario)

Preparation: 15 minutes
Cook: 5 minutes
Makes 6 servings

Calories per serving: 74
Grams of protein per serving: 5.3
Grams of fat per serving: 2.9
Grams of carbohydrate per serving: 8.6
Grams of fibre per serving: 3.3

Iceberg lettuce will keep fresh longer if you store it properly. It should be cored and washed first. Store lettuce away from fruits like melons or apples, as they give off ethylene gas. This gas can cause rust spotting on the lettuce.

GARDEN COTTAGE CHEESE SALAD
Susan Close, Kitchener, Ontario

The zing of Dijon mustard in this recipe will awaken your taste buds.

1½ cups	low-fat (2 percent) cottage cheese	375 mL
¾ cup	diced English cucumber	175 mL
½ cup	shredded carrot	125 mL
½ cup	shredded zucchini	125 mL
1	green onion, chopped	1
2 tsp.	Dijon mustard	10 mL
¼ tsp.	Worcestershire sauce	1 mL
	Lettuce leaves or whole wheat pitas or tomatoes	

In bowl, combine cottage cheese, cucumber, carrot, zucchini, onion, and seasonings. Cover and chill to blend flavours.

Serve as a main course salad on lettuce; as a sandwich filling in a pita pocket; or use as a stuffing for hollowed-out tomatoes.

Variation: Prepare as an appetizer by stuffing the mixture into cherry tomatoes or hollowed out cucumber chunks.

Preparation: 15 minutes
Chill: 1 hour or longer
Makes 4 servings

Calories per serving: 88
Grams of protein per serving: 11.9
Grams of fat per serving: 1.8
Grams of carbohydrate per serving: 6.0
Grams of fibre per serving: 0.8

CARROT AND ORANGE SALAD WITH YOGHURT

Judy Koster, Bridgewater, Nova Scotia

Quick and simple to prepare, this salad can be served with cold or barbecued meats. Peach yoghurt can be replaced with other fruit-flavoured yoghurts for a change.

1½ cups	grated carrot	375 mL
½ cup	orange sections	125 mL
½ cup	raisins	125 mL
⅓ cup	coarsely chopped walnuts	75 mL
¼ cup	low-fat peach yoghurt	50 mL
1 tsp.	lemon juice	5 mL
1 tsp.	granulated sugar	5 mL
¼ tsp.	salt	1 mL
	Lettuce leaves	

In medium bowl, combine carrot and orange sections. Pour boiling water over raisins to cover. Let stand 5 minutes and drain; add to carrot mixture. Stir in walnuts, yoghurt, lemon juice, sugar, and salt. To serve, spoon on lettuce leaves.

MENU SUGGESTION

This moist and delicious salad provides fibre and vitamin A. The yoghurt dressing keeps the fat content low. Serve it with Inge-leoge Vis (page 47), California Casserole (page 165), and fresh fiddleheads with lemon for a protein-rich meal. For a satisfying finish, prepare Winter Fruit Crisp (page 222). (Kathleen Hodgins, R.D., Thompson, Manitoba)

Preparation: 10 minutes
Chill: 30 minutes or longer
Makes 4 to 6 servings

Calories per serving: 106
Grams of protein per serving: 2.1
Grams of fat per serving: 3.5
Grams of carbohydrate per serving: 18.7
Grams of fibre per serving: 2.2

VARIETY GREENS WITH FRESH STRAWBERRIES

Janice McDowell, Penticton, British Columbia

The wide assortment of interesting salad greens inspires creativity in salad making. Try the relatively new red leaf lettuce, the pungent arugula, and peppery watercress as well as the more common greens such as bibb or iceberg lettuce. A refreshing salad that even when served with Raspberry Basil Vinaigrette contains only one gram of fat per serving.

DRESSING

¼ cup	fresh orange juice	50 mL
1 tbsp.	fresh lemon juice	15 mL
1 tbsp.	chopped fresh mint	15 mL
1 tsp.	granulated sugar	5 mL
½ tsp.	grated orange peel	2 mL
¼ tsp.	grated lemon peel	1 mL
1 cup	sliced strawberries	250 mL

4 cups	assorted lettuce, torn into bite-sized pieces	1 L
½ cup	sliced red onion	125 mL
½ cup	alfalfa sprouts	125 mL

In salad bowl, combine lettuce, onion, and sprouts; cover and refrigerate.

Combine orange and lemon juice, mint, sugar, and peel. Pour over sliced strawberries; cover and refrigerate.

Just before serving, pour strawberry mixture over salad greens; toss gently.

Variation: Canned, drained Mandarin oranges may replace strawberries.

Alfalfa and bean sprouts are no longer just a food of the flower-child generation. Some sprouts are getting hot. Sprout growers are sprouting radish and mustard seeds. These sprouts have a hot, piquant flavour. Read the label on the sprout packages to find the hot sprouts. Try them in salads or even as a topping for a hot dog or hamburger.

Preparation: 15 minutes
Chill: about 30 minutes
Makes 6 servings

Calories per serving: 23
Grams of protein per serving: 0.7
Grams of fat per serving: 0.2
Grams of carbohydrate per serving: 5.2
Grams of fibre per serving: 1.1

HAWAIIAN CRANBERRY SALAD
Carol Sage, Scarborough, Ontario

This moulded salad is an excellent accompaniment to a poultry dinner. For a buffet party, the recipe may be doubled.

1 cup	boiling water	250 mL
1	package (85 g) orange-flavoured gelatine	1
1	can (6.5 oz./184 mL) whole cranberry sauce	1
1 cup	crushed pineapple with juice	250 mL
½ cup	chopped celery	125 mL
	Garnish: orange slices, parsley, lettuce leaves	

In small bowl, pour boiling water over gelatine; stir until dissolved. Stir in cranberry sauce, pineapple, and celery. Pour into a rinsed 4-cup (1 L) mould; cover and refrigerate until firm, about 3 hours.

To serve, unmould on serving plate; garnish with orange slices and parsley or lettuce.

Preparation: 15 minutes
Chill: about 3 hours
Makes 6 servings

Calories per serving: 132
Grams of protein per serving: 1.6
Grams of fat per serving: 0.1
Grams of carbohydrate per serving: 33.0
Grams of fibre per serving: 0.6

HOT AND SPICY FRUIT SLAW
Marlyn Ambrose-Chase, Moose Jaw, Saskatchewan

This unusual hot cabbage salad has the spicy flavour of Indian curries. Curry lovers may want to increase the amount of curry powder.

1	small green cabbage	1
⅓ cup	finely chopped green onion	75 mL
¼ cup	finely chopped celery	50 mL
3 tbsp.	butter or margarine	45 mL
1 to 2 tsp.	curry powder	5 to 10 mL
1 tsp.	corn starch	5 mL
¼ tsp.	salt	1 mL
Pinch	freshly ground black pepper	Pinch
1 cup	orange juice	250 mL
1	carrot, thinly sliced	1
1	red cooking apple, cut into wedges	1
2	oranges, peeled and sectioned	2
¼ cup	chutney	50 mL

Remove 4 to 6 outer cabbage leaves; blanch in boiling water until slightly wilted, about 15 seconds. Rinse under cold water; drain well and set aside.

Slice remaining cabbage into very thin strips.

In large skillet over medium-high heat, cook onion and celery in butter for about 3 minutes. Stir in curry powder, cornstarch, salt, and pepper; cook, stirring frequently for 5 minutes. Stir in orange juice, sliced cabbage, and carrots. Cover and bring to boil; reduce heat and cook for 10 minutes.

Add apple; cook, stirring, about 2 minutes. Stir in oranges and chutney; heat thoroughly for about 4 minutes. Serve in large bowl lined with blanched cabbage leaves.

MENU SUGGESTION

This hot cabbage salad provides a delicious source of vitamins A and C as well as fibre. Serve it with tandoori chicken, herbed potatoes, and whole wheat pita bread, followed by frozen berry yoghurt for a nutritious meal that meets Canada's Food Guide. (Kelly McQuillen, Whitehorse, Yukon)

Preparation: 25 minutes
Cook: approximately 15 minutes
Makes 6 servings

Calories per serving: 161
Grams of protein per serving: 2.3
Grams of fat per serving: 6.1
Grams of carbohydrate per serving: 27.3
Grams of fibre per serving: 4.8

TARRAGON VINAIGRETTE POTATO SALAD

Donna Nadolny, Brampton, Ontario

A vinaigrette dressing is a refreshing change from the traditional mayonnaise-dressed potato salad. Coarse grainy mustard and tarragon gives this old favourite a new and tangy twist.

> Since vinegar removes colour from radish skin, add sliced radish just before serving.
>
> Do not economize too much when buying red wine vinegar. Buy a good-quality product, which will enhance the flavour of this recipe.

MENU SUGGESTION

This salad is a lower-fat version of the traditional potato salad. This dressing keeps the fat low and the potatoes provide complex carbohydrates and fibre. Serve it alongside salmon steaks with lemon wedges and Lightly Glazed Stir-Fried Vegetables (page 120), and prepare fresh fruit with yoghurt dressing for dessert. (Ellen Vogel, R.D., Winnipeg, Manitoba)

Preparation: 20 minutes
Chill: 1 hour or longer
Makes 6 servings

Calories per serving: 107
Grams of protein per serving: 2.3
Grams of fat per serving: 2.5
Grams of carbohydrate per serving: 20.0
Grams of fibre per serving: 2.3

3	large potatoes, unpeeled	3
2 tbsp.	red wine vinegar	25 mL
1 tbsp.	vegetable oil	15 mL
1	small clove garlic, minced	1
2 tsp.	dried tarragon	10 mL
1 tsp.	coarse grainy mustard	5 mL
½ tsp.	horseradish	2 mL
¼ tsp.	salt	1 mL
¼ tsp.	freshly ground pepper	1 mL
½ cup	sliced celery	125 mL
¼ cup	sliced green onion	50 mL
¼ cup	chopped yellow pepper	50 mL
½ cup	thinly sliced radish	125 mL
	Garnish: celery leaves	

Cook potatoes in boiling water until tender; drain and partially cool. Cut into cubes. Whisk together vinegar, oil, garlic, and seasonings. Pour dressing over warm potatoes. Cover and refrigerate until cool.

Add celery, onion, and yellow pepper to potato mixture. Cover and refrigerate for at least 1 hour before serving. Add radish, garnish with celery leaves, and serve.

GOLDEN TREASURE SALAD
Betty Dent, Belleville, Ontario

This colourful salad can easily be served all year round. It is best when made ahead and refrigerated.

DRESSING

1 cup	low-fat plain yoghurt	250 mL
¼ cup	liquid honey	50 mL
3 tbsp.	lemon juice	45 mL

1	small bunch broccoli, chopped (about 2 cups/500 mL)	1
1 cup	grated carrots	250 mL
1 cup	sunflower seeds	250 mL
1 cup	raisins	250 mL
2	green onions, chopped	2

In large bowl, combine broccoli, carrots, sunflower seeds, raisins, and onion.

Combine yoghurt, honey, and lemon juice. Pour dressing over vegetables; toss until well coated. Cover and refrigerate 1 to 2 hours.

MENU SUGGESTION

The sunflower seeds in this recipe are nutritious but high in fat, so serve this salad with a low-fat meal. Try it with salmon poached in white wine with herbs, confetti rice, and steamed green beans with nutmeg. Orange sherbet makes a light dessert. (Louise Poole, Yellowknife, Northwest Territories)

Preparation: 15 minutes
Chill: 1 to 2 hours
Makes 6 servings

Calories per serving: 303
Grams of protein per serving: 10.1
Grams of fat per serving: 12.4
Grams of carbohydrate per serving: 44.8
Grams of fibre per serving: 5.2

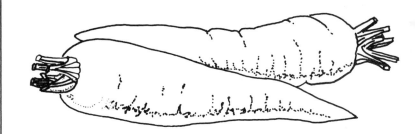

WINTER VEGETABLE SALAD
Betty Jane Humphrey, Owen Sound, Ontario

Prepare this satisfying recipe when lettuces and other salad vegetables are more expensive.

DRESSING

¼ cup	low-fat plain yoghurt	50 mL
1 tbsp.	cider vinegar	15 mL
1 tbsp.	chili sauce	15 mL
1 tsp.	horseradish	5 mL
Pinch	salt	Pinch

½ lb.	parsnips, cut into ½-inch (2-cm) chunks	225 g
½ lb.	carrots, cut into ½-inch (2-cm) chunks	225 g
2	stalks celery, sliced	2
½	small red onion, chopped	½
½ cup	raisins	125 mL

Steam parsnips and carrots over boiling water until crisp-tender. Rinse under cold water and drain well. In medium bowl, combine parsnips, carrots, celery, red onion, and raisins.

Combine yoghurt, vinegar, chili sauce, horseradish, and salt. Pour dressing over vegetables; mix until well coated. Cover and refrigerate at least 1 hour.

Preparation: 15 minutes
Cook: 10 to 15 minutes
Chill: 1 hour
Makes 4 to 6 servings

Calories per serving: 106
Grams of protein per serving: 2.2
Grams of fat per serving: 0.5
Grams of carbohydrate per serving: 25.3
Grams of fibre per serving: 3.7

BROWN RICE À L'ORANGE SALAD
Fran J. Maki, Surrey, British Columbia

This excellent brown rice and fruit salad gained honourable mention in the final judging of the Healthy Eating recipe contest.

DRESSING

¼ cup	light mayonnaise	50 mL
3 tbsp.	orange juice concentrate	45 mL
3 tbsp.	vegetable oil	45 mL
1 tbsp.	lemon juice	15 mL
1 tbsp.	liquid honey	15 mL
¼ tsp.	dry mustard	1 mL
⅛ tsp.	Tabasco sauce	0.5 mL

¾ cup	brown rice	175 mL
2 cups	boiling water	500 mL
¾ cup	sliced celery	175 mL
1	can (10 oz./284 mL) mandarin oranges, drained	1
½ cup	pineapple chunks	125 mL
12	sliced, pitted black olives	12
2 tbsp.	sunflower seeds	25 mL
	Garnish: lettuce leaves, whole strawberries, sunflower seeds	

In saucepan, add rice to boiling water. Cover and cook 45 minutes, or until tender and water is absorbed. Cool.

In medium bowl, combine rice, celery, oranges, pineapple, black olives, and sunflower seeds.

Combine mayonnaise, orange juice, oil, lemon juice, honey, and seasonings. Pour over salad; stir gently to mix. Cover and refrigerate 1 hour.

Line 6 plates with lettuce leaves. Spoon rice mixture into centre; garnish with strawberries and sunflower seeds.

MENU SUGGESTION

This colourful salad provides vitamin C, B vitamins, and fibre. However, some of the ingredients are high in fat, so trim the overall fat content of the meal by serving cold barbecued chicken with the skin removed, whole wheat rolls, and Piquant Marinated Vegetables (page 48). Round out the meal with fresh berries. (Patti Benzer, R.D.N., Kelowna, British Columbia)

Preparation: 10 minutes
Cook: 40 to 45 minutes
Chill: 1 hour
Makes 6 servings

Calories per serving: 289
Grams of protein per serving: 3.6
Grams of fat per serving: 13.0
Grams of carbohydrate per serving: 41.7
Grams of fibre per serving: 2.5

SPINACH AND RICE SALAD
Gertrude Boudreau, Rockland, Ontario

A favourite recipe with the panel! You'll want to keep the dressing on hand for other salads, so make the entire recipe and refrigerate the leftover.

DRESSING

½ cup	vinegar	125 mL
½ cup	granulated sugar	125 mL
2 tsp.	lemon juice	10 mL
1 tsp.	chopped fresh parsley	5 mL
1 tsp.	dry mustard	5 mL
Pinch	paprika, cayenne, garlic powder, salt, and pepper	Pinch
1 cup	olive oil	250 mL

¾ cup	long grain white rice	175 mL
2 cups	boiling water	500 mL
¼ cup	olive oil	50 mL
2 tbsp.	soy sauce	25 mL
1 cup	bean sprouts	250 mL
1 cup	torn spinach leaves	250 mL
½ cup	chopped green pepper	125 mL
¼ cup	raisins	50 mL
2 tbsp.	chopped fresh parsley	25 mL
2 tbsp.	chopped green onion	25 mL

In saucepan, add rice to boiling water. Cover and cook 20 minutes, or until tender and water is absorbed. Add oil and soy sauce; allow to cool.

In large bowl, combine rice mixture, bean sprouts, spinach, green pepper, raisins, parsley, and onion.

Whisk together, vinegar, sugar, lemon juice, parsley, mustard, and seasonings. Gradually whisk in oil. Pour ¼ cup (50 mL) dressing over salad. Refrigerate remaining dressing for other salads.

MENU SUGGESTION

Serve this salad with herbed lemon lamb chops, julienne carrots, and Whole Wheat Biscuits (page 190). To keep the fat in control, broil the lamb chops, steam the carrots, and use a very small amount of butter on the biscuits. Finish the meal with Strawberry Sorbet (page 223). (Christine Williams, R.P.Dt., Belleville, Ontario)

Preparation: 10 minutes
Cook: 20 to 25 minutes
Makes about 1½ cups (375 mL) of dressing; 6 servings of salad

Calories per serving: 257
Grams of protein per serving: 3.3
Grams of fat per serving: 14.7
Grams of carbohydrate per serving: 29.1
Grams of fibre per serving: 1.2

JELLIED GAZPACHO SALAD
Marie Hermary, Red Deer, Alberta

A new twist on the classic Mexican soup. All the zesty flavours of gazpacho prepared as a jellied salad. It is loaded with crunch but light on fat. Enjoy it any time you are looking for a cool salad.

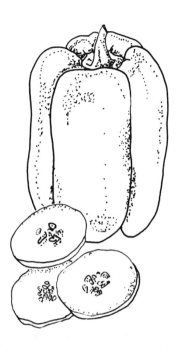

1	envelope unflavoured gelatine	1
1¼ cups	vegetable juice cocktail, divided	300 mL
1 tsp.	beef bouillon powder	5 mL
2 tbsp.	cider vinegar or white vinegar	25 mL
1 tsp.	Worcestershire sauce	5 mL
Dash	hot pepper sauce	Dash
1	medium tomato, peeled	1
½	large green pepper	½
½	large cucumber, peeled and seeded	½
1	small onion	1
1	small clove garlic	1
1	small celery stalk with leaves	1
	Garnish: celery leaves	

Preparation: 15 minutes
Cook: 3 minutes
Chill: 3 hours
Makes 6 servings

Calories per serving: 31
Grams of protein per serving: 2.0
Grams of fat per serving: 0.3
Grams of carbohydrate per serving: 6.2
Grams of fibre per serving: 0.9

In medium saucepan, sprinkle gelatine over ¼ cup (50 mL) vegetable juice. Stir over low heat for 3 minutes, or until gelatine is completely dissolved. Stir in beef bouillon, ¾ cup (175 mL) vegetable juice, vinegar, Worcestershire sauce, and hot pepper sauce. Refrigerate, stirring occasionally, until mixture is consistency of unbeaten egg whites, about 30 minutes.

In food processor or blender, purée half the tomato, green pepper, cucumber, onion, and garlic with remaining vegetable juice until smooth. Coarsely chop remaining tomato and celery. Stir purée and chopped vegetables into gelatine mixture. Pour into a rinsed 6 cup (1.5 L) mould. Cover and refrigerate until firm, at least 3 hours.

To serve, unmould gazpacho onto serving plate. Garnish with celery leaves.

CREATE YOUR OWN PASTA SALAD
Janice Dillman, Dartmouth, Nova Scotia

The panel loved this pasta salad with its many variations. Try rotini, fusilli, elbow macaroni, or shells in plain or coloured pasta. Cooked chicken, tuna, or salmon may be added to make this into a main course salad.

DRESSING

⅓ cup	white vinegar or cider vinegar	75 mL
1 tsp.	prepared mustard	5 mL
½ tsp.	garlic powder	2 mL
½ tsp.	dried thyme	2 mL
½ tsp.	dried oregano	2 mL
Dash	Worcestershire sauce	Dash
3 tbsp.	canola oil or safflower oil	45 mL

3 cups	cooked pasta	750 mL
2 cups	diced raw vegetables (any combination of green pepper, radish, cauliflower, broccoli, carrot, green onion, and celery)	500 mL

In large bowl, combine pasta and raw vegetables. Whisk together vinegar and seasonings. Gradually whisk in oil. Pour over pasta mixture. Cover and refrigerate for 1 hour.

MENU SUGGESTION

The amount of oil makes this salad higher in fat, so use the dressing sparingly and accompany the salad with low-fat choices. Try it with Beef Barley Soup (page 71), Super Health Bread (page 189), marinated tomatoes, and skim milk. (Susan Close, R.P.Dt., Kitchener, Ontario)

Preparation: 15 minutes
Chill: 1 hour
Makes 6 servings

Calories per serving: 178
Grams of protein per serving: 3.7
Grams of fat per serving: 8.4
Grams of carbohydrate per serving: 22.9
Grams of fibre per serving: 1.8

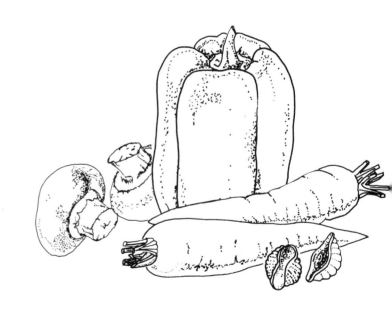

SALADE À LA GOUT

Elaine L. Ginbey, Nanaimo, British Columbia

This attractive salad combines lettuce with chick peas, and red pepper in a low-fat yoghurt dressing. Prepare ahead and toss with lettuce just before serving.

DRESSING

⅓ cup	low-fat plain yoghurt	75 mL
1 tsp.	lemon juice	5 mL
1 tbsp.	chopped fresh parsley	15 mL
1 tbsp.	chopped fresh chives	15 mL
1 tbsp.	chopped fresh dill or	15 mL
1 tsp.	dried dill	5 mL
1	large clove garlic, crushed	1

1	medium head lettuce	1
1	can (14 oz./398 mL) chick peas, drained	1
1	red pepper, quartered and sliced	1
¼ cup	sunflower seeds	50 mL

Tear lettuce into bite-sized pieces. In large salad bowl, combine lettuce, chick peas, red pepper, and sunflower seeds.

Combine yoghurt, lemon juice, parsley, chives, dill, and garlic. Pour dressing over lettuce; toss until well coated.

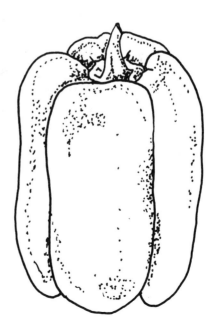

MENU SUGGESTION

This salad can be served either as a side dish or as an entrée. Complement the protein in the chick-peas with the protein in Super Health Bread (page 189). Round out the meal with a milky Berry Shake (page 239) that isn't too high in fat. (Barb Colvin, P.Dt., Regina, Saskatchewan)

Preparation: 15 minutes
Makes 6 servings

Calories per serving: 124
Grams of protein per serving: 5.9
Grams of fat per serving: 3.9
Grams of carbohydrate per serving: 17.6
Grams of fibre per serving: 4.0

TABBOULEH

Johanne Trudeau, Oakville, Ontario

Mint and lemon are the traditional flavours found in this classic Middle Eastern salad. Unlike most salads, this one is best made ahead and refrigerated. Be sure to serve this with Falafel (page 111).

DRESSING

¼ cup	lemon juice	50 mL
3 tbsp.	olive oil	45 mL
1	small clove garlic, minced	1
½ tsp.	grated lemon peel	2 mL
½ tsp.	granulated sugar	2 mL
½ tsp.	dry mustard	2 mL
¼ tsp.	paprika	1 mL
¼ tsp.	salt	1 mL
	Freshly ground pepper	

1 cup	medium-grain bulgur (cracked wheat)	250 mL
1 cup	boiling water	250 mL
5 to 6	green onions, chopped	5 to 6
1½ cups	lightly packed parsley sprigs	375 mL
⅓ cup	lightly packed fresh mint leaves	75 mL
2	tomatoes, chopped	2

In covered saucepan, cook bulgur in boiling water for about 5 minutes, or until liquid is absorbed (bulgur should still be crunchy). Turn into a large bowl; allow to cool.

In food processor, coarsely chop onions, parsley, and mint leaves; add to bulgur. Stir in tomatoes.

Whisk together lemon juice, olive oil, garlic, lemon peel, sugar, and seasonings. Pour dressing over bulgur mixture; mix together lightly. Cover and refrigerate for several hours or overnight.

> To keep parsley and mint fresh, store in tightly covered container in refrigerator.

Preparation: 15 minutes
Cook: 5 minutes
Chill: several hours
Makes 6 cups (1.5 L) or about 8 servings

Calories per serving: 135
Grams of protein per serving: 3.3
Grams of fat per serving: 5.4
Grams of carbohydrate per serving: 19.9
Grams of fibre per serving: 2.9

WEST COAST CHICKEN SALAD
Fran J. Maki, Surrey, British Columbia

Serve this salad as a main course for a light summer meal. It is a Canadian adaptation of a fresh fruit tropical salad; however, tropical fruit like fresh pineapple may be used. Use the same dressing with other fruit salads.

DRESSING

¼ cup	vinegar	50 mL
3 tbsp.	liquid honey	45 mL
2 tbsp.	lime juice	25 mL
1 tsp.	poppy seeds	5 mL
¼ tsp.	dry mustard	1 mL
½ cup	safflower oil	125 mL

3 ½ cups	cooked, cubed chicken	875 mL
	Lettuce leaves	
½	honeydew melon, peeled and cut into wedges or balls	½
1	small cantaloupe, peeled and cut into wedges or balls	1
1 ¼ cups	sliced strawberries	300 mL
1 cup	green grapes	250 mL
½ cup	blueberries	125 mL

Whisk together vinegar, honey, lime juice, poppy seeds, and dry mustard. Gradually whisk in oil.

Place chicken in large bowl. Pour all but ⅓ cup (75 mL) dressing over chicken, tossing to mix; reserve remaining dressing. Cover and refrigerate chicken for 1 hour.

To serve, arrange lettuce, honeydew, and cantaloupe on 6 chilled plates. Spoon chicken mixture into centre of each. Toss remaining dressing with strawberries, grapes, and blueberries. Spoon fruit mixture on each salad.

With fresh pineapple, consider a garnish of pineapple leaves.

MENU SUGGESTION

This attractive salad provides protein, vitamin C, and fibre. However, the safflower oil in the dressing is the primary source of fat, so use it sparingly. Serve it with Apricot Bran Bread (page 202), and Icy Yoghurt Pops (page 213) for dessert. (Tracy Darychuck, R.D.N., Westminster, British Columbia)

Preparation: 20 minutes
Chill: 1 hour
Makes 6 servings

Calories per serving: 426
Grams of protein per serving: 24.2
Grams of fat per serving: 24.1
Grams of carbohydrate per serving: 31.2
Grams of fibre per serving: 2.5

SUPER SALMON SALAD
Kraft General Foods

This salad combines cooked pasta—use the coloured version, if available—vegetables, Swiss cheese, and salmon with a light, lower-calorie, lower-fat, commercial cucumber dressing. When it is served on a bed of spinach leaves, you will enjoy this eye-catching main course salad.

1 cup	coloured fusilli	250 mL
1 ½ cups	frozen peas, thawed and drained	375 mL
¼ cup	diced Swiss cheese	50 mL
1	can (3.75 oz./106 g) red salmon, drained, broken into chunks	1
½ cup	grated carrot	125 mL
½ cup	light creamy cucumber dressing	125 mL
	Spinach leaves, stems removed	

Cook pasta according to package directions; drain. To cool quickly, rinse under cold water; drain well. Combine pasta, peas, Swiss cheese, salmon, carrot, and cucumber dressing; toss lightly. Refrigerate covered until ready to serve on spinach-lined plates.

MENU SUGGESTION

This salad contains all four food groups in one dish. For additional fibre, serve it with a pumpernickel roll, Tropical Fruit Slush (page 239), and Peachy Upside-Down Cake (page 208). (Mary Sue Waisman, R.D., Calgary, Alberta)

Preparation: 15 minutes
Cook: 10 to 15 minutes
Makes 3 to 4 servings

Calories per serving: 286
Grams of protein per serving: 14.3
Grams of fat per serving: 9.9
Grams of carbohydrate per serving: 34.4
Grams of fibre per serving: 3.5

Photos: West Coast Chicken Salad, page 151 (facing page); Country Club Pasta, page 174 (overleaf)

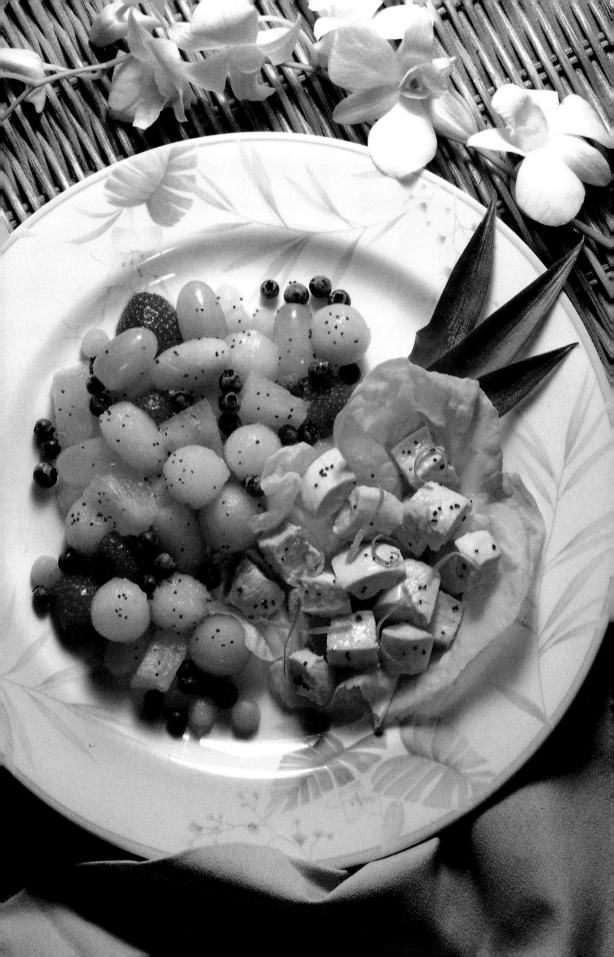

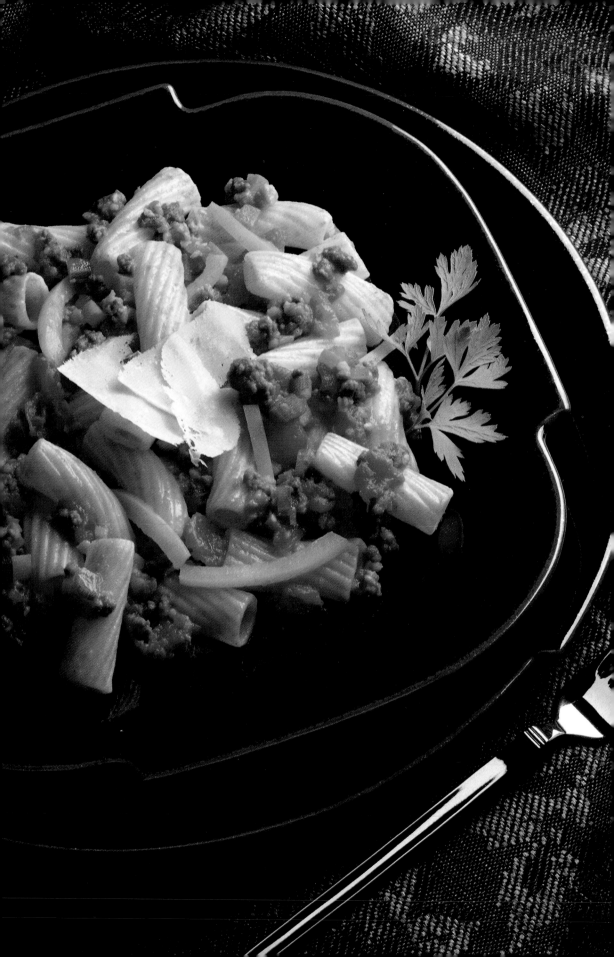

Radicchio is a trendy type of lettuce that is small in size but often big on price. This red and white lettuce, originally from Italy, resembles an oversized brussels sprout. Its flavour is pleasantly sharp. The individual leaves are a perfect size to hold an appetizer. As well, a little bit of radicchio in a green salad will give it a special flavour and colour.

RASPBERRY BASIL VINAIGRETTE
Erna Braun, Winnipeg, Manitoba

Most salad greens perk up with a special dressing using interesting vinegars. Raspberry, balsamic, tarragon vinegars — all add extra zest to dressings.

½ cup	water	125 mL
2 tbsp.	raspberry vinegar	25 mL
1	small clove garlic, crushed	1
1 tsp.	cornstarch	5 mL
1 tsp.	olive oil	5 mL
1 tsp.	fresh basil or	5 mL
½ tsp.	dried basil	2 mL
½ tsp.	poppyseeds	2 mL
¼ tsp.	grated lemon or orange peel	1 mL
Pinch	salt	Pinch

To make your own raspberry vinegar, add fresh or frozen raspberries to rice or white wine vinegar; let stand at room temperature for several days. Strain and bottle.

In small saucepan, cook water, vinegar, garlic, and cornstarch for about 2 minutes, or until thickened. Allow to cool. In small bowl, combine oil, basil, poppyseeds, lemon peel, and salt. Stir in vinegar mixture; cover and refrigerate for at least 1 hour.

Preparation: 10 minutes
Chill: about 1 hour
Makes ½ cup (125 mL)
Serving size: 1 tbsp./15 mL

Calories per serving: 8
Grams of protein per serving: 0
Grams of fat per serving: 0.6
Grams of carbohydrate per serving: 0.7
Grams of fibre per serving: 0

SESAME VINAIGRETTE
The Canadian Dietetic Association

Enjoy this citrus salad dressing over your favourite greens: Boston lettuce, radicchio, curly or Belgian endive. Add fresh herbs like parsley, dill, oregano, or basil, and slivers of Swiss, Cheddar, Muenster, or Emmenthal cheese.

Preparation: 5 minutes
Makes about ⅓ cup (75 mL)
Serving size: 1 tbsp./15 mL

Calories per serving: 18
Grams of protein per serving: 0.7
Grams of fat per serving: 1.1
Grams of carbohydrate per serving: 1.4
Grams of fibre per serving: 0

¼ cup	low-fat plain yoghurt	50 mL
2 tbsp.	grapefruit juice	25 mL
1 tsp.	sesame oil	5 mL
¼ tsp.	salt	1 mL
¼ tsp.	pepper	1 mL

In blender, combine yoghurt, grapefruit juice, oil, and seasonings. Blend on low speed for 30 seconds.

HERB TOMATO SALAD DRESSING
Ellen Vogel, Winnipeg, Manitoba

You will want to serve this refreshing no-fat dressing over tasty, crisp greens or drizzled over sliced cucumber.

Red wine vinegar is better in this recipe than malt or cider vinegar because it is closer in flavour to the traditional French vinaigrette dressing.

Preparation: 5 minutes
Chill: 1 hour or longer
Makes 1 cup (250 mL)
Serving size: 1 tbsp./15 mL

Calories per serving: 5
Grams of protein per serving: 0.2
Grams of fat per serving: 0
Grams of carbohydrate per serving: 1.3
Grams of fibre per serving: 0

1	can (7 ½ oz./213 mL) tomato sauce	1
2 tbsp.	red wine vinegar	25 mL
1 tsp.	Worcestershire sauce	5 mL
1 tsp.	Italian seasoning	5 mL
½ tsp.	dried dill weed	2 mL
Pinch	freshly ground pepper	Pinch
1	green onion, thinly sliced	1

In jar, combine tomato sauce, vinegar, and seasonings. Cover and shake well; add green onion. Refrigerate for at least 1 hour for best flavour development.

BLUE CHEESE SALAD DRESSING
Ann Roberts, Maple Ridge, British Columbia

The tanginess of this dressing will enhance a tossed green salad or a lettuce wedge. It also may be used as a dip for raw vegetables or fresh fruits.

Preparation: 5 minutes
Chill: 1 hour or longer
Makes ¾ cup (175 mL)
Serving size: 1 tbsp./15 mL

Calories per serving: 47
Grams of protein per serving: 3.0
Grams of fat per serving: 3.4
Grams of carbohydrate per serving: 1.1
Grams of fibre per serving: 0

½ cup	low-fat plain yoghurt	125 mL
1 cup	crumbled blue cheese	250 mL
1 tbsp.	2 percent milk	15 mL
1	clove garlic, crushed	1

In food processor or blender, blend yoghurt, blue cheese, milk, and garlic until smooth. Refrigerate until serving time.

LEMON PESTO DRESSING
Margaret Howard, Toronto, Ontario

Keep a supply of Lemon Pesto Sauce (page 177) on hand to make this and many other recipes.

Makes about 1 cup (250 mL)
Serving size: 1 tbsp./15 mL

Calories per serving: 25
Grams of protein per serving: 0.3
Grams of fat per serving: 2.3
Grams of carbohydrate per serving: 0.9
Grams of fibre per serving: 0.2

¼ cup	light mayonnaise	50 mL
½ cup	buttermilk	125 mL
3 tbsp.	Lemon Pesto Sauce (page 177)	45 mL

Combine mayonnaise, buttermilk, and sauce. Keep refrigerated. Serve over your favourite salad greens.

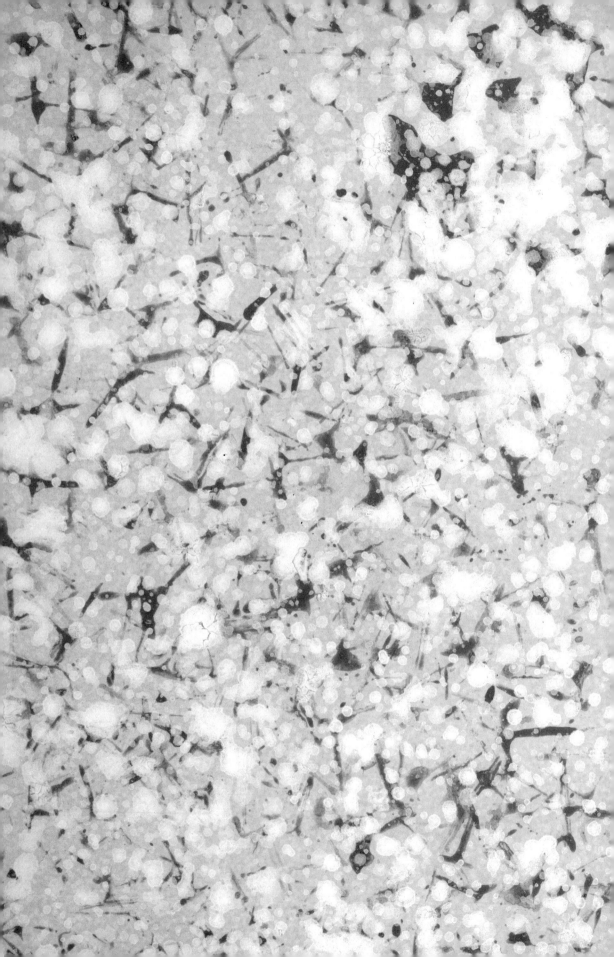

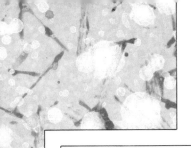

RICE, PASTA, AND GRAINS

We hope this section will introduce you to a few new foods in the grains category: quinoa (a seed-like grain), barley flakes (an important cereal), and millet (the smallest size of cracked wheat, used to make porridge and a North African dish called couscous). Other grains — like bulgur, or cracked wheat, which is used for Tabbouleh (page 150), and comes in several different sizes, and brown rice — are now readily available in supermarkets.

PASTA PATTER: Let's talk about the many varieties of pasta. There are 325 different shapes, with 50 commonly found on store shelves. The most popular varieties are spaghetti, spaghettini, macaroni, lasagna, and all sizes of noodles.

Many stores now carry fresh pasta in the refrigerator cases. Most people think it tastes better than dried. It certainly cooks faster — usually in 3 to 4 minutes — but it will not keep for more than 2 or 3 days in the refrigerator. Freeze for longer storage. Dried pasta requires longer cooking — usually 3 to 4 times as long as fresh, depending on the shape — but it has a longer shelf life.

What about enriched pasta? Enrichment is a process that puts back most of the major vitamins and minerals that were removed through milling. Whole wheat pasta is made from whole wheat flour and has a small increase in fibre and B vitamins.

What about coloured and flavoured pastas? These pastas are now available, especially as fresh, in a wide variety of flavours: basil, sage, tarragon, red pepper, tomato, shrimp, black (squid ink), lemon, even chocolate (for chocoholics), as well as the more common spinach. The extra ingredients primarily add colour and some flavour — with little or no extra nutrition.

HOW TO COOK PASTA

The biggest danger is over-cooking. If the pot is too small and you do not use enough water, invariably the pasta will be gummy. The ideal pot is both wide and deep. You can never go wrong by using too much water, even when cooking a small amount of pasta.

Be sure water is boiling hard before adding pasta. It is unnecessary to add salt, but 1 tsp. (5 mL) oil helps to keep the pasta from sticking to the pot and itself. After the pasta has been added, keep the water at a full rolling boil. Stir once or twice after first adding to pot. Always leave the pot uncovered. Cook pasta according to package directions, or until it is *al dente* (tender but firm). Drain, don't rinse pasta, unless you are not using it right away. Then, rinse the drained pasta to prevent it from sticking together.

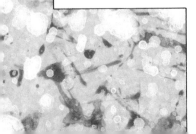

RICE SAVVY

Rice has been referred to as "the pasta of the 1990s." Annual consumption of rice in Canada doubled in the last decade, partly as a result of the introduction to our diets of European and Asian rice dishes.

The best-known and most frequently used rices are long- or short-grain white rice, converted rice, and instant rice. Brown rice is gaining in popularity. It contains B vitamins and trace minerals, as well as incomplete protein. It has a decidedly stronger flavour than white. When possible, choose brown over white. Rice bran, found in brown rice, is also a source of soluble fibre. Wild rice, which is not a rice at all but a grass, is rather expensive and used generally in small quantities with other types of rice. It has similar nutrients to brown—protein, B vitamins, and iron. New to our culinary world are two ancient rice varieties, referred to as the aromatic rices. Basmati rice, with its appealing aroma and subtle flavour, is used in Mixed Rice Casserole (page 168) and arborio rice is used for Italian Risotto (page 161).

Long-grain rice, traditionally preferred in Canada, cooks dry, fluffy, and separate. Short-grain, the rice of choice in parts of the Orient and in Mediterranean countries, is moist, clingy (sticky), and soft after cooking, and is very well suited to rice puddings. Start watching for jasmine, texmati, wild pecan, and wehani rices, which will be appearing in the next few years.

LET'S COOK RICE

	WHITE Long Grain	WHITE Short Grain	BROWN RICE	BASMATI RICE	WILD RICE
Amount (Raw)	1 cup (250 mL)	1 cup (250 mL)	1 cup (250 mL)	1 cup (250 mL)	½ cup (125 mL)
Water	2 cups (500 mL)	1¼ cups (300 mL)	3 cups (750 mL)	2 cups (500 mL)	2 cups (500 mL)
Cook	15 to 20 minutes	15 to 20 minutes	45 minutes	15 to 20 minutes	40 to 45 minutes
Yield (Cooked)	3 cups (750 mL)	3 cups (750 mL)	3 cups (750 mL)	3 cups (750 mL)	2 cups (500 mL)
Servings	4 to 5	4 to 5	4 to 5	4 to 5	3 to 4

COOKING RICE

Bring water to a boil. Add rice, return to boil. Cook, covered, on medium-low heat for required time, or until little holes appear in the surface of the rice and all liquid is absorbed. Do not peek during cooking!

RICE SOUFFLÉ
Ethel St. Jean, New Liskeard, Ontario

Glamorous soufflés are considered difficult, but really are easy. This soufflé uses shortcuts – leftover cooked rice and a can of cream of mushroom soup.

½ cup	chopped onion	125 mL
1 tbsp.	butter or margarine	15 mL
1 tsp.	curry powder	5 mL
1	can (10 oz./284 mL) condensed cream of mushroom soup	1
1 cup	shredded old Cheddar cheese	250 mL
6	eggs, separated	6
1½ cups	cooked white rice (½ cup/125 mL uncooked long-grain white rice)	375 mL

In skillet on medium heat, cook onion in butter until softened; stir in curry powder, soup, and Cheddar cheese. Heat slowly until cheese melts; stir occasionally. Beat egg yolks thoroughly and stir into hot soup mixture. Stir in cooked rice.

In large bowl, beat egg whites until stiff but not dry. With spatula, lightly fold egg whites into rice mixture. Turn into an ungreased 8-cup (2 L) casserole. Bake at 300°F (150°C) for about 1 hour, or until soufflé is golden brown and knife inserted in centre of puff comes out clean. Do not open oven door during first 20 minutes of baking.

MENU SUGGESTION

This delicate rice soufflé provides complex carbohydrates, protein, iron, and calcium, but gets a large proportion of its calories from fat. Reduce the meal's overall fat content by serving it with a tossed green salad, whole wheat mini bagels, broccoli spears, and carrot coins. Finish the meal with a citrus fruit salad. (Wanda Smith-Windsor, R.D., Selkirk, Manitoba)

Preparation: 10 minutes
Cook: about 1 hour
Makes 6 servings

Calories per serving: 273
Grams of protein per serving: 12.6
Grams of fat per serving: 17.6
Grams of carbohydrate per serving: 15.6
Grams of fibre per serving: 0.4

Canadians are enjoying mushrooms more today than a generation ago. We're eating 700 percent more mushrooms now than in 1963. Even so, that is only about two and a half pounds of fresh mushrooms per person a year. To get the best flavour and nutrition from your mushrooms, rinse and pat them dry just before eating. Don't scrub or peel them; it results in nutrient loss and a change in texture.

RICE PILAF

Marilyn Peters, Martintown, Ontario

Mushrooms, almonds, and raisins give this savoury rice pilaf an interesting blend of flavours. Use a homemade chicken broth or a low-salt chicken bouillon powder. Since brown rice requires about 45 minutes cooking time, you may need to watch that it does not boil dry.

½ cup	raisins	125 mL
¼ cup	slivered almonds	50 mL
2 tbsp.	butter or margarine, divided	25 mL
1 cup	brown rice	250 mL
1	small onion, chopped	1
2	cloves garlic, minced	2
2½ cups	chicken broth	625 mL
1	bay leaf	1
2 tbsp.	lemon juice	25 mL
1 tsp.	grated lemon rind	5 mL
Dash	freshly ground pepper	Dash
1 cup	sliced mushrooms	250 mL

In saucepan on medium heat, cook raisins and almonds in 1 tbsp. (15 mL) butter until golden; reserve.

In same saucepan on medium-high heat, cook rice, onion, and garlic in 1 tbsp. (15 mL) butter for 5 minutes, or until light brown. Add chicken broth, bay leaf, lemon juice, lemon rind, and pepper. Cover and cook on low heat for 40 minutes. Add mushrooms; cook 5 minutes. Remove bay leaf. Serve rice sprinkled with reserved raisins and almonds.

MENU SUGGESTION

This recipe is an interesting way to "fancy up" your rice. The fibre comes primarily from the brown rice, raisins, and nuts. The nuts also contribute a substantial proportion of the fat. Serve with Cheesy Salmon Loaf (page 89), steamed asparagus with calorie-reduced dressing, a multi-grain roll, and fruit with yoghurt dressing. (Rosario Soneff, R.D.N., Penticton, British Columbia)

Preparation: 10 minutes
Cook: 45 minutes
Makes 6 servings

Calories per serving: 263
Grams of protein per serving: 6.8
Grams of fat per serving: 8.1
Grams of carbohydrate per serving: 42.2
Grams of fibre per serving: 3.5

ITALIAN RISOTTO
Brenda Sledzinski, Calgary, Alberta

The creamy texture of Italian risotto is obtained by slowly adding chicken broth during the cooking process to a short-grain rice called arborio. Risotto can be served as a one-dish main course with the addition of cooked meat and vegetables, or as a side dish.

4 cups	chicken broth	1 L
¼ cup	finely chopped onion	50 mL
1 tbsp.	olive oil	15 mL
¼ cup	dry white wine	50 mL
1 cup	arborio rice or Italian short-grain rice	250 mL
3 tbsp.	freshly grated Parmesan cheese	45 mL
	Freshly ground pepper	

During addition of chicken broth, be careful to stir gently so rice kernels do not break up and become mushy. It is helpful to set a timer for 22 minutes when you add first quantity of chicken broth.

In large covered saucepan, bring chicken broth to a boil.

Meanwhile, in large saucepan on medium heat, cook onion in oil for about 5 minutes, or until tender but not browned; stir frequently. Stir in rice, cook until all grains are coated, about 1 minute. Add wine and cook until almost evaporated. Add ½ cup (125 mL) hot chicken broth.

Cook, stirring gently with a wooden spoon, until almost all liquid has been absorbed. Continue adding chicken broth in ½ cup (125 mL) amounts until all broth has been used; stir constantly. This technique will require about 22 minutes total cooking time. The rice will be creamy, moist, and *al dente* (tender but firm). Remove from heat; stir in Parmesan cheese. Add freshly ground pepper to taste.

Preparation: 10 minutes
Cook: about 22 minutes
Makes 6 servings

Calories per serving: 131
Grams of protein per serving: 5.6
Grams of fat per serving: 3.9
Grams of carbohydrate per serving: 17.6
Grams of fibre per serving: 0.6

RICE PIZZA
Cathy Hatch, Edmonton, Alberta

Brown rice provides an excellent crust for this vegetarian pizza. The tomato sauce and brown rice may be cooked ahead. Makes two pizzas; you can freeze one for later use.

TOPPINGS

1½ cups	thinly sliced mushrooms	375 mL
1 cup	thinly sliced zucchini	250 mL
1	small green pepper, diced	1
1	medium tomato, chopped	1
½ cup	broccoli florets	125 mL
½ cup	cauliflower florets	125 mL
1½ cups	shredded low-fat mozzarella cheese	375 mL

CRUST

1 cup	brown rice	250 mL
3 cups	boiling water	750 mL
1 cup	grated low-fat mozzarella cheese	250 mL
2	eggs, beaten	2
½ tsp.	dry mustard	2 mL
Dash	pepper	Dash

SAUCE

¼ cup	minced onion	50 mL
1	clove garlic, minced	1
1 tbsp.	vegetable oil	15 mL
1	can (14 oz./398 mL) crushed tomatoes	1
1 tbsp.	chopped fresh parsley or	15 mL
1 tsp.	dried parsley	5 mL
½ tsp.	dried basil	2 mL
½ tsp.	dried oregano	2 mL
½ tsp.	granulated sugar	2 mL

MENU SUGGESTION

This pizza is almost a complete meal in itself. For added appeal, serve with a spinach salad and a whole grain roll. Lemon Pudding (page 232) makes a tangy dessert. (Barb Colvin, P.Dt., Regina, Saskatchewan)

In covered saucepan, add rice to boiling water. Cover and cook on low for 45 minutes, or until rice is tender and water is absorbed; cool. Combine rice, cheese, eggs, and seasonings. Press mixture into 2 lightly greased 9-inch (23

Preparation: 45 minutes
Cook: 20 to 25 minutes
Makes two 9-inch (23-cm) pizzas or 8 servings

Calories per serving: 258
Grams of protein per serving: 14.0
Grams of fat per serving: 9.7
Grams of carbohydrate per serving: 29.6
Grams of fibre per serving: 3.4

cm) pie plates. Bake in 450°F (230°C) oven for about 10 minutes.

Meanwhile, prepare sauce: In skillet on medium-high heat, cook onion and garlic in oil for about 5 minutes, or until softened. Add tomatoes, seasonings, and sugar. Simmer, uncovered, about 20 minutes, or until thickened.

Spread sauce over rice crust. Top with mushrooms, zucchini, green pepper, tomato, broccoli, and cauliflower. Sprinkle with cheese. Bake in 400°F (200°C) oven for about 20 minutes.

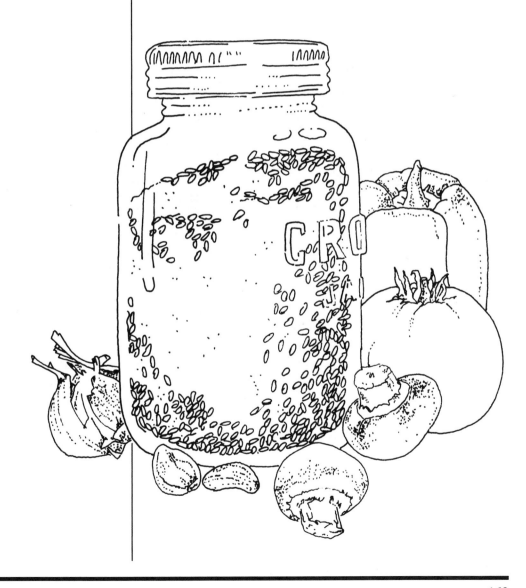

A MEAL-IN-ONE
Karen Quinn, Arkona, Ontario

Microwave casseroles are extremely handy on busy days.

½ cup	chopped onion	125 mL
½ cup	chopped celery	125 mL
2 tbsp.	butter or margarine	25 mL
2 cups	cooked chicken, cut into bite-size pieces	500 mL
1¾ cups	hot water	425 mL
⅔ cup	long-grain white rice	150 mL
1	can (10 oz./284 mL) mushrooms, undrained	1
1 cup	frozen peas and carrots	250 mL
½ tsp.	dried thyme	2 mL
½ tsp.	dried rosemary	2 mL

MENU SUGGESTION

This is a hearty dish that is economical and easy to prepare. Since it contains ingredients from all the four food groups, a glass of milk is all that is needed to complete the meal. Serve with a multigrain roll and a green garden salad with Herb Tomato Salad Dressing (page 154) for extra fibre and vitamins. Round out the meal with cantaloupe and lime sherbet. (Jean Norman, R.Dt., St. John's, Newfoundland)

Microwave Method: Combine onion, celery, and butter in 8-cup (2-L) microwavable dish. Microwave, covered, on High (100 percent) for 5 minutes. Stir in chicken, water, rice, mushrooms, peas, and carrots, and seasonings. Microwave on High for 6 minutes, then microwave on Medium (50 percent) for 10 to 12 minutes, or until rice is tender and most of the water has been absorbed. Let stand for 10 minutes before serving.

Oven Method: In skillet, cook onion and celery in butter until soft. Stir in remaining ingredients. Bake in covered casserole, in 350°F (180°C) oven for about 30 minutes or until rice is cooked.

Preparation: 10 minutes
Microwave: about 20 minutes
Makes 4 servings

Calories per serving: 285
Grams of protein per serving: 22.7
Grams of fat per serving: 10.8
Grams of carbohydrate per serving: 23.7
Grams of fibre per serving: 3.3

CALIFORNIA CASSEROLE
Lauren Forsyth, The Pas, Manitoba

Casseroles like this rice one can be frozen to serve on a busy day.

MENU SUGGESTION

When you select this recipe, you need to control the fat in your other choices. To increase the fibre content, try using brown or wild rice. Serve with Ingeleoge Vis (page 47), Carrot and Orange Salad with Yoghurt (page 138), fresh fiddleheads with lemon, and Winter Fruit Crisp (page 222) for a meal that meets Canada's Food Guide. (Kathleen Hodgins, R.D., Thompson, Manitoba)

¾ cup	long-grain white rice	175 mL
2 cups	water	500 mL
1 cup	light sour cream	250 mL
1 cup	shredded medium Cheddar cheese	250 mL
½ cup	low-fat (2 percent) cottage cheese	125 mL
½ cup	chopped onion	125 mL
¼ cup	chopped mushrooms	50 mL
¼ cup	chopped green pepper	50 mL
½ tsp.	salt	2 mL
¼ tsp.	freshly ground pepper	1 mL

In large saucepan, add rice to boiling water. Cover and cook on low for about 20 minutes, or until rice is tender and water is absorbed. Let stand 5 minutes.

Combine hot rice, sour cream, Cheddar and cottage cheese, onion, mushrooms, green pepper, and seasonings. Turn into a lightly greased 6-cup (1.5-L) casserole. Bake, uncovered, in 350°F (180°C) oven for about 25 minutes.

Preparation: 15 to 20 minutes
Cook: 25 minutes
Makes 6 servings

Calories per serving: 220
Grams of protein per serving: 10.4
Grams of fat per serving: 9.4
Grams of carbohydrate per serving: 22.8
Grams of fibre per serving: 0.6

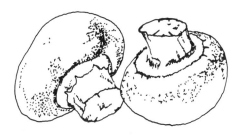

WILD RICE AND STIR-FRY VEGETABLE DISH

Ethel Sorokowsky, Edmonton, Alberta

This colourful side dish combines broccoli, cauliflower, carrots, red pepper, green beans, and mushrooms with two kinds of rice—brown and wild. Add extra soy sauce for more of an oriental flavour. If you are following a vegetarian diet, use vegetable bouillon instead of chicken bouillon, or replace all liquid with tomato juice or vegetable juice cocktail.

1¼ cups	water	300 mL
2 tsp.	chicken bouillon	10 mL
½ tsp.	dried thyme	2 mL
¼ cup	wild rice	50 mL
¼ cup	brown rice	50 mL
2 tbsp.	canola oil	25 mL
¼ cup	slivered almonds	50 mL
1½ cups	cut-up green beans	375 mL
1 cup	broccoli florets	250 mL
1 cup	cauliflower florets	250 mL
1 cup	sliced carrots	250 mL
1 cup	sliced mushrooms	250 mL
¼ cup	sliced red pepper	50 mL
¼ cup	chopped green onion	50 mL
1 tbsp.	soy sauce	15 mL
2 tsp.	lemon juice	10 mL
½ tsp.	grated lemon rind	2 mL

In large saucepan on high heat, bring water, chicken bouillon, and thyme to a boil. Add wild and brown rice. Cover and cook on low for about 45 minutes, or until rice is tender.

MENU SUGGESTION

The rices and vegetables in this dish combine to provide a good source of complex carbohydrates and fibre. Serve with steamed filet of sole, followed by fresh fruit and skim milk. (MaryAnne Zupancic, R.D.N., Nanaimo, British Columbia)

Preparation: 15 minutes
Cook: 45 minutes
Makes 4 to 5 servings

Calories per serving: 201
Grams of protein per serving: 6.5
Grams of fat per serving: 9.6
Grams of carbohydrate per serving: 25.0
Grams of fibre per serving: 5.1

In large skillet on medium-high, heat oil. Add almonds and cook for about 2 minutes, or until golden brown. Remove and set aside. To skillet add green beans, broccoli, cauliflower, carrots, mushrooms, and red pepper; stir-fry for about 5 minutes. Add 2 tbsp. (25 mL) water. Cover and steam for 3 minutes. Remove cover; add green onion. Cook on high, stirring constantly, to evaporate excess liquid. Add soy sauce, lemon juice, and rind. Toss to combine.

Arrange cooked rice on platter; spoon vegetables over rice and sprinkle with reserved almonds.

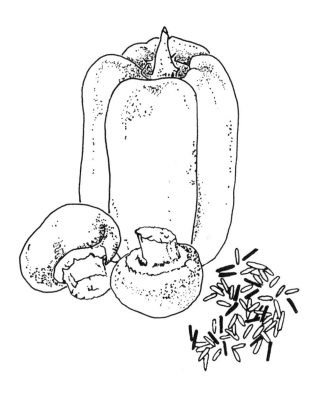

MIXED RICE CASSEROLE
Selma Savage, Toronto, Ontario

This mixture of fragrant basmati and wild rice with brightly coloured vegetables will liven up any dinner. The Indian seasonings may be increased, if desired. For variety, add garnishes of mandarin oranges and pistachio nuts.

Basmati rice is considered the best of the long-grained rices. It is becoming more widely available in supermarkets, but can always be found in health food stores. It is best known for its fragrant aroma and flavour.

¼ cup	wild rice	50 mL
3 cups	boiling water, divided	750 mL
1 cup	basmati rice	250 mL
2	carrots, chopped	2
2	celery stalks, chopped	2
1	medium onion, chopped	1
½	red pepper, chopped	½
½	green pepper, chopped	½
1	clove garlic, minced	1
2 tbsp.	vegetable oil	25 mL
3 tbsp.	soy sauce	45 mL
¼ tsp.	dried cumin	1 mL
¼ tsp.	dried coriander	1 mL
¼ tsp.	dried oregano	1 mL
¼ tsp.	curry powder	1 mL
Dash	chili powder	Dash
¼ cup	shelled sunflower seeds	50 mL

MENU SUGGESTION

The fat in this recipe comes from the oil and seeds. Balance it out with lower-fat accompaniments. Add protein to the meal with Tangy Glazed Chicken (page 80) and fibre with pea pods and Cinnamon Baked Pears (page 219). (Sharon Cazakoff, P.Dt., Regina, Saskatchewan)

Preparation: 45 minutes
Cook: 4 to 5 minutes
Makes 6 servings

Calories per serving: 192

Wash wild rice under cold running water; drain well. Add rice to 1 cup (250 mL) boiling water. Cover and cook on low for 45 minutes, or until rice is tender but firm. Drain well.

Meanwhile, in large saucepan, add basmati rice to remaining boiling water. Cover and cook on low for about 20 minutes, or until rice is tender and water is absorbed. Let stand 5 minutes.

Just before both rices have finished cooking, cook

Grams of protein per serving: 4.9

Grams of fat per serving: 7.5

Grams of carbohydrate per serving: 27.3

Grams of fibre per serving: 2.4

carrots, celery, onion, peppers, and garlic in large skillet in oil for 4 to 5 minutes, or until crisp-tender. Stir in soy sauce and seasonings.

Combine vegetable mixture with hot cooked wild and basmati rice; sprinkle with sunflower seeds.

ITALIAN-STYLE MACARONI

Liliane Cotton, Gaspé, Quebec

The tomato sauce for this macaroni is cooked to reduce the volume. The sauce will be thin when added to the macaroni, but will thicken during the oven baking. If desired, Parmesan could replace Cheddar cheese.

MENU SUGGESTION

This macaroni dish provides fewer calories and less fat than conventional macaroni and cheese. Using low-fat cheese decreases the fat content even further. Serve with lean back bacon for protein and broiled zucchini, carrot sticks, and celery stalks for fibre and vitamins. Finish the meal with a fruit salad. (Adele Harrison, R.P.Dt., Red Lake, Ontario)

Preparation: 25 minutes

Cook: 25 to 30 minutes

Makes 4 servings

Calories per serving: 240

Grams of protein per serving: 12.4

Grams of fat per serving: 10.2

Grams of carbohydrate per serving: 25.2

Grams of fibre per serving: 0.6

2 cups	tomato juice	500 mL
1 cup	chicken broth	250 mL
2 tbsp.	finely chopped onion	25 mL
1	clove garlic, minced	1
1 tsp.	Italian herb seasoning	5 mL
Pinch	salt and pepper	Pinch
2 cups	cooked elbow macaroni	500 mL
1 cup	shredded old Cheddar cheese	250 mL

In medium saucepan, combine tomato juice, broth, onion, garlic, and seasonings. Cook, uncovered, for about 25 minutes, or until reduced in half.

Stir tomato sauce into cooked macaroni. Turn into medium-sized baking pan. Sprinkle with cheese. Bake in 375°F (190°C) oven for about 25 minutes.

TUNA GARDEN
Karen B. Wall, Whitby, Ontario

Tuna Garden was another favourite recipe of our taste panelists. The light sauce, prepared with chicken broth for the pasta, allows the vegetables and tuna to be featured. For variety, use whole wheat spaghetti.

MENU SUGGESTION
This recipe provides abundant protein, fibre, vitamins, and iron, with minimal fat. Serve with garlic bread, a lettuce wedge with vinaigrette, and gingerbread with lemon sauce. (Cheryl Rayter, R.D., Winnipeg, Manitoba)

6	large mushrooms, sliced	6
1	small onion, sliced	1
2 tbsp.	butter or margarine	25 mL
2	cans (each 6.5 oz./184 g) chunk white tuna, packed in water, drained	2
2 cups	chicken broth	500 mL
2 tbsp.	all-purpose flour	25 mL
2 tbsp.	lemon juice	25 mL
2 tbsp.	chopped pimento	25 mL
1 tsp.	grated lemon rind	5 mL
1 tsp.	dried thyme	5 mL
¼ tsp.	garlic powder	1 mL
Dash	salt and pepper	Dash
3	medium carrots, sliced	3
2	large stalks broccoli (florets only), chopped	2
½ lb.	spaghettini noodles	250 g
	Garnish: tomato slices	

Preparation: 15 minutes
Cook: 10 to 12 minutes
Makes 6 servings

Calories per serving: 310
Grams of protein per serving: 25.9
Grams of fat per serving: 5.4
Grams of carbohydrate per serving: 39.1
Grams of fibre per serving: 3.8

In large skillet on medium heat, cook mushrooms and onion in butter for about 5 minutes, or until tender. Stir in tuna. Combine chicken broth, flour, lemon juice, pimento, lemon rind, and seasonings. Stir into tuna mixture; cook for about 5 minutes, or until slightly thickened.

Steam carrots and broccoli over boiling water until crisp-tender. Drain well and add to tuna mixture.

In large pot of boiling water, cook noodles according to package directions, or until *al dente* (tender but firm); drain well. Stir tuna and vegetable sauce into noodles; garnish with tomato slices.

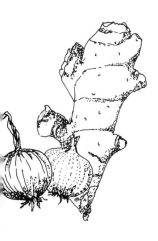

GINGER LINGUINE
Paul Howard, Kingston, Ontario

While a student at Queen's University, Paul Howard made this easily prepared, yet unusual dish for classmates at dinner parties. Beware, there is spice and heat; it is not for the timid! For a change, try grated Romano in place of the Parmesan.

½ lb.	linguine	250 g
2 tbsp.	chopped gingerroot	25 mL
3	large cloves garlic, minced	3
2 tbsp.	butter or margarine	25 mL
1 tbsp.	chopped fresh basil	15 mL
	or	
1 tsp.	dried basil	5 mL
1 tsp.	hot pepper sauce	5 mL
3	green onions, finely chopped	3
	Freshly ground pepper	
¼ cup	grated Parmesan cheese	50 mL
	Garnish: chopped fresh basil	

If you use the narrower pastas, like linguine and spaghettini, the sauce will stick to the pasta rather than be left behind in the pot.

Preparation: 15 minutes
Cook: 10 to 15 minutes
Makes 4 servings

Calories per serving: 290
Grams of protein per serving: 9.6
Grams of fat per serving: 7.7
Grams of carbohydrate per serving: 45.0
Grams of fibre per serving: 1.6

In large pot of boiling water, cook linguine according to package directions, or until *al dente* (tender but firm). Drain well.

Meanwhile, in large skillet on medium-high heat, cook gingerroot and garlic in butter until softened, about 2 minutes. Add basil, pepper sauce, green onions, and pepper to taste; cook about 2 minutes (be sure onions do not wilt).

Toss drained linguine with sauce and cheese until well coated; garnish with fresh basil. Serve immediately.

PASTA WITH BROCCOLI HERB SAUCE
Tanis Fenton, Calgary, Alberta

This broccoli sauce is similar to a Basil Pesto Sauce and is intended to be thick. However, if you want a thinner sauce, chicken stock may be added. Serve over fettucine, fusilli, or linguine. What a great way for the kids to eat their broccoli!

MENU SUGGESTION

This unique sauce made from pur-eed broccoli is rich in fibre and vitamin C. Serve with skinless roast chicken breasts, raw carrot sticks, and skim milk for a bal-anced meal and finish with straw-berries for dessert. (Melanie Reeves, R.D., Calgary, Alberta)

2¾ cups	chopped broccoli	675 mL
⅓ cup	olive or vegetable oil	75 mL
⅓ cup	grated Parmesan cheese	75 mL
¼ cup	chopped fresh parsley or	50 mL
1 tbsp.	dried parsley	15 mL
1 tbsp.	fresh basil or	15 mL
1 tsp.	dried basil	5 mL
¾ lb.	pasta	400 g

Preparation: 10 minutes
Microwave: 4 to 5 minutes
Cook: 10 to 12 minutes (dry pasta), 4 to 5 minutes (fresh pasta)
Makes 4 to 5 main course servings; 8 to 10 appetizer servings

Calories per serving as a main course: 422

Grams of protein per serving: 13.3

Grams of fat per serving: 16.3

Grams of carbohydrate per serving: 56.5

Grams of fibre per serving: 4.1

Calories per serving as an appetizer: 211

Grams of protein per serving: 6.6

Grams of fat per serving: 8.2

Grams of carbohydrate per serving: 28.2

Grams of fibre per serving: 2.1

Place broccoli and 2 tbsp. (25 mL) water in 4-cup (1 L) microwavable bowl. Microwave, covered, on High (100 percent) for about 5 minutes; drain.

In food processor, purée broccoli, oil, cheese, parsley, and basil until broccoli is finely chopped.

Cook pasta in boiling water according to package directions, or until *al dente* (tender but firm). Drain well and toss with vegetable mixture. Serve immediately.

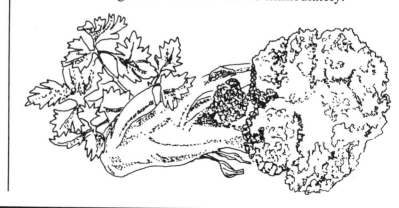

GARDEN FETTUCINE

Kathy Sziklai, Vancouver, British Columbia

This light-flavoured sauce will remind you of garden-fresh vegetables.

1 cup	finely chopped onion	250 mL
2	cloves garlic, minced	2
2 tbsp.	olive oil	25 mL
3 cups	peeled and chopped tomatoes	750 mL
3 tbsp.	fresh basil leaves, chopped or	45 mL
2 tsp.	dried basil	10 mL
1	zucchini, diced	1
½ lb.	fettucine	250 g
	Garnish: chopped fresh basil (optional), Parmesan cheese	

In large skillet on medium heat, cook onion and garlic in oil until softened, about 5 minutes. Add tomatoes and basil and simmer for about 10 minutes, or until slightly thickened. Add zucchini and cook for 2 minutes.

In large pot of boiling water, cook fettucine according to package directions, or until *al dente* (tender but firm). Drain well.

Combine sauce and fettucine until well coated; sprinkle with chopped fresh basil (if using) and cheese. Serve immediately.

MENU SUGGESTION

The tomato sauce in this pasta dish is lower in calories and fat than a cream-based sauce. For a summer evening meal, serve with barbecued seafood kebabs and a salad of butter lettuce and mushrooms with vinaigrette and toasted almonds. Seasonal fresh fruit with ice milk makes a refreshing dessert. This provides calcium, vitamins, and minerals. (Jeanne McCutcheon, R.D.N., Richmond, British Columbia)

Preparation: 10 minutes
Cook: 10 to 15 minutes
Makes 4 servings

Calories per serving: 323
Grams of protein per serving: 9.8
Grams of fat per serving: 7.7
Grams of carbohydrate per serving: 55.4
Grams of fibre per serving: 4.6

COUNTRY CLUB PASTA

Linda Terra, Calgary, Alberta

This delicious new dish for pasta lovers combines meat and vegetables in a delectable sauce. For a zestier sauce, add dried basil, oregano, and rosemary.

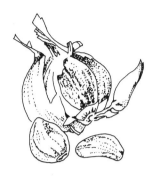

2	yellow peppers, cut into slices	2
2 tbsp.	vegetable oil or olive oil	25 mL
1	small onion, chopped	1
1	small carrot, chopped	1
1	celery stalk, chopped	1
1	large clove garlic, minced	1
¼ lb.	lean ground beef	125 g
1	can (14 oz./398 mL) tomatoes	1
½ tsp.	salt	2 mL
¼ tsp.	freshly ground pepper	1 mL
2 oz.	cooked ham, finely chopped	50 g
1	package (300 g) penne pasta	1
½ cup	grated Parmesan cheese	125 mL
	Garnish: parsley sprigs	

In skillet over medium-high heat, cook peppers in oil for about 3 minutes; set aside.

In medium saucepan, cook onion, carrot, celery, garlic, and ground beef until meat loses pink colour; drain fat. Add tomatoes, and seasonings. Cook, uncovered, over medium-low heat for 15 minutes. Stir in pepper slices and ham; cook about 15 minutes, or until thickened.

In large pot of boiling water, cook pasta according to package directions, or until *al dente* (tender but firm). Drain well.

Toss meat sauce and pasta until well coated. Sprinkle with cheese; garnish with parsley. Serve immediately.

MENU SUGGESTION

Served with Italian bread and a crisp tossed salad, this pasta is the basis of a meal that's low in fat and sodium and rich in calcium, iron, vitamin A, and dietary fibre. Round out the meal with fresh cherries for dessert. (Elizabeth Farrell, P.Dt., Saint John, New Brunswick)

Preparation: 30 minutes
Cook: 15 to 20 minutes
Makes 4 servings

Calories per serving: 494
Grams of protein per serving: 23.4
Grams of fat per serving: 15.0
Grams of carbohydrate per serving: 65.7
Grams of fibre per serving: 3.8

Roasted or grilled sweet peppers have a rich, smoky flavour with a firm texture. To roast, prick the pepper with a fork and place it in a hot oven. Cook until the pepper skin is blistered. Then place the pepper in a paper or plastic bag, close it, and let the pepper sweat for about 10 minutes. The skin will slip off quite easily.

EASY SAILING LUNCH
Gwen Sawchuk, Edmonton, Alberta

The Sawchuk family prepared this recipe frequently for lunch while on a sailing holiday in the Greek Islands and served it with pork chops and green beans. Orzo pasta is available in some grocery stores, health food stores, and specialty food shops.

½	small red pepper, chopped	½
½	large onion, chopped	½
1	clove garlic, chopped	1
2 tbsp.	olive oil	25 mL
1 cup	orzo pasta	250 mL
1	medium tomato, chopped	1
	Salt and pepper to taste	

In skillet on medium-high heat, cook red pepper, onion, and garlic in oil until tender, about 5 minutes.

Cook pasta in boiling water about 10 minutes, or until *al dente* (tender but firm). Drain well and toss with vegetable mixture.

Stir in tomato and seasonings. Serve immediately.

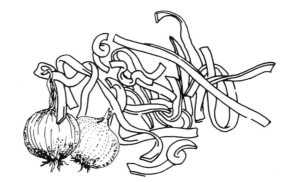

Preparation: 10 minutes
Cook: 10 to 15 minutes
Makes 4 to 6 servings

Calories per serving: 170
Grams of protein per serving: 4.5
Grams of fat per serving: 4.8
Grams of carbohydrate per serving: 26.9
Grams of fibre per serving: 1.2

VERSATILE TOMATO SAUCE
Brenda Steinmetz, Toronto, Ontario

With a can of tomatoes, a few vegetables, and seasonings, this thick tomato-rich sauce, a traditional pasta favourite, is quickly prepared. Use it for pizza, over cooked pasta, for canneloni, lasagna, or Lasagna Roll-ups (page 106).

At the peak of the tomato harvest, you can replace the canned tomatoes in this recipe with 8 to 10 peeled ripe tomatoes. You may need to cook the sauce longer, depending on the amount of liquid in the tomatoes. Make one batch or several, and freeze for later use.

1	medium onion, chopped	1
½ cup	chopped celery	125 mL
½ cup	shredded carrot or zucchini	125 mL
½ cup	chopped green pepper	125 mL
1	clove garlic, chopped	1
1 tsp.	vegetable oil	5 mL
1	can (28 oz./796 mL) tomatoes	1
¼ cup	red wine	50 mL
1	bay leaf	1
½ tsp.	dried oregano	2 mL
½ tsp.	dried basil	2 mL
¼ tsp.	salt	1 mL
¼ tsp.	pepper	1 mL
¼ tsp.	dried parsley	1 mL
Pinch	cinnamon (optional)	Pinch

Preparation: 15 minutes
Cook: about 1 hour
Makes about 3 cups (750 mL) or 5 to 6 servings

Calories per half cup (125 mL) of sauce: 48

Grams of protein per serving: 1.7

Grams of fat per serving: 1.2

Grams of carbohydrate per serving: 9.0

Grams of fibre per serving: 1.9

In large saucepan on medium-high heat, cook onion, celery, carrot, green pepper, and garlic in oil, stirring frequently for about 10 minutes, or until tender. Stir in tomatoes, red wine, and seasonings.

Cook on medium heat, uncovered, for about 1 hour, or until thickened; stir frequently. Remove bay leaf before serving.

Variations
MEAT SAUCE
Add ½ lb. (250 g) lean ground beef, browned or shaped into small meatballs to Versatile Tomato Sauce.

RED CLAM SAUCE
Add 1 can clams, undrained, to Versatile Tomato Sauce.

STUFFED PEPPERS
Stuff peppers with cooked rice; bake topped with Versatile Tomato Sauce.

CABBAGE ROLLS
Pour Versatile Tomato Sauce over cabbage rolls.

CHICKEN MARENGO
Replace red wine in Versatile Tomato Sauce with white wine and add sliced mushrooms. Cook chicken pieces in this sauce.

MEATLOAF
Serve sliced meatloaf with Versatile Tomato Sauce.

LEMON PESTO SAUCE
Margaret Howard, Toronto, Ontario

This concentrated pesto sauce is the basis for several other recipes. Keep a supply in the freezer. For a more traditional pesto, you may wish to replace almonds with pine nuts.

* When fresh basil is not available, replace with 1 cup (250 mL) fresh parsley leaves and 2 tbsp. (25 mL) dried basil. As well, spinach leaves are another replacement for fresh basil.

Makes ⅓ cup (75 mL).
Preparation: 15 minutes
Chill or freeze: as desired

Calories per tablespoon: 40
Grams of protein per tablespoon: 0.7
Grams of fat per tablespoon: 3.6
Grams of carbohydrate per tablespoon: 2.0
Grams of fibre per serving: 0.2

1 cup	packed fresh basil leaves*	250 mL
1	clove garlic	1
1 tbsp.	olive oil	15 mL
1 tbsp.	almonds or pine nuts	15 mL
4 tsp.	fresh lemon juice	20 mL
1 tsp.	grated lemon rind	5 mL

In food processor or blender, combine basil, garlic, oil, almonds, lemon juice, and rind. Blend until coarsely chopped.

Pasta sauce: Combine Lemon Pesto Sauce and grated Parmesan cheese; toss with pasta or egg noodles for a traditional Italian meal.

CORNMEAL CASSEROLE
Lydia Husak, Calgary, Alberta

Cornmeal is made from ground corn and is a great source of complex carbohydrates.

MENU SUGGESTION

For an inexpensive meatless meal, complement Cornmeal Casserole with Stir-Fried Vegetables with Tofu (page 110) and sliced cucumbers with vinaigrette. The protein in the corn and the tofu combine to provide a high-quality meatlike protein with plenty of fibre. Round out the meal with low-fat yoghurt and fresh berries. (Mary Sue Waisman, R.D., Calgary, Alberta)

1	small onion, chopped	1
1	stalk celery, chopped	1
1 tbsp.	butter or margarine	15 mL
½ cup	yellow cornmeal	125 mL
½ tsp.	salt	2 mL
½ tsp.	granulated sugar	2 mL
Dash	freshly ground pepper	Dash
2 cups	2 percent milk	500 mL
1	egg, well beaten	1

In skillet on medium heat, cook onion and celery in butter until golden. Stir in cornmeal and mix until coated. Add salt, sugar, and pepper.

Scald milk; stir into cornmeal mixture. Cook on low heat until thickened; allow to cool. Stir in beaten egg and mix well. Turn mixture into a lightly greased 4-cup (1-L) casserole. Bake, uncovered, in 350°F (180°C) oven for 35 to 40 minutes, or until top is browned and casserole is set.

Preparation: 10 minutes
Cook: 35 to 40 minutes
Makes 4 servings

Calories per serving: 170
Grams of protein per serving: 6.9
Grams of fat per serving: 6.6
Grams of carbohydrate per serving: 20.4
Grams of fibre per serving: 1.2

Broccoli and cauliflower broken into flowerets have about half the shelf life of those left whole.

VEGETABLE QUINOA
Monique Clément, Gloucester, Ontario

Quinoa (pronounced keen-wa) is a seed-like grain available from health food stores which originates from the Andes Mountains in South America. It was one of the three staple foods, along with corn and potatoes, of the Inca civilization. Serve with your favourite meat.

1 cup	quinoa	250 mL
1 cup	boiling water	250 mL
¼ cup	diced tomatoes	50 mL
¼ cup	carrot strips	50 mL
¼ cup	chopped broccoli	50 mL
¼ cup	cauliflower florets	50 mL
¼ cup	diced zucchini	50 mL
2 tbsp.	sunflower oil	25 mL
1 tbsp.	soy sauce	15 mL

Rinse quinoa under cold water until water runs clear. In medium saucepan, add quinoa to boiling water, cover, and simmer for about 15 minutes, or until tender. (Watch carefully to prevent sticking.)

In skillet on medium-high heat, stir-fry tomatoes, carrot, broccoli, cauliflower, and zucchini in oil for about 4 minutes. Stir vegetables and soy sauce into quinoa and serve immediately.

MENU SUGGESTION

Quinoa provides a new twist to a stir-fry with its slightly crunchy texture and nutty flavour. Serve a chicken vegetable stir-fry with quinoa for high-quality protein as well as vitamins and minerals. Add won ton soup for an unusual meal. Fresh or frozen raspberries with low-fat yoghurt provide a refreshing source of additional fibre. (Barbara Burton, R.P.Dt., Gloucester, Ontario)

Preparation: 10 minutes
Cook: 15 minutes
Makes 6 servings

Calories per serving: 164
Grams of protein per serving: 4.8
Grams of fat per serving: 6.1
Grams of carbohydrate per serving: 25.0
Grams of fibre per serving: 0.6

GRANOLA

Denise A. Hartley, Calgary, Alberta

This is probably one of the best granola recipes you will ever make!
Enjoy as a cereal, with yoghurt, over fruit, or as a snack.

5 cups	large-flake rolled oats	1.25 L
2 cups	barley flakes	500 mL
1½ cups	raw unsalted nuts (almonds, filberts, pecans), chopped	375 mL
1 cup	sesame seeds	250 mL
1 cup	raw, unsalted, shelled sunflower seeds	250 mL
1 cup	raw, unsalted pumpkin seeds	250 mL
1 cup	skim-milk powder	250 mL
1 cup	wheat germ	250 mL
1 cup	unsweetened coconut	250 mL
¾ cup	olive oil or canola oil	175 mL
½ cup	molasses	125 mL
½ cup	liquid honey	125 mL
1 tbsp.	cinnamon	15 mL
2 cups	dried fruit (raisins, apricots, mango, pineapple, banana), cut up	500 mL

In large roasting pan, mix oats, barley flakes, raw nuts, sesame, sunflower, and pumpkin seeds, skim-milk powder, wheat germ, and coconut.

Combine oil, molasses, honey, and cinnamon. Stir thoroughly into oat mixture.

Bake in 325°F (160°C) oven for about 30 minutes, or until golden brown; stir frequently. Allow to cool; stir in fruit. Store, covered, in a cool, dry location.

MENU SUGGESTION

This granola is great for an energy-packed breakfast. Like most granolas, however, it is high in fat and calories, so keep the rest of the meal low in fat. Serve with skim milk or yoghurt and a fresh fruit cup made of ½ banana, ½ orange, and ¼ cup fresh or frozen berries. (Deborah Leach, R.Dt., St. John's, Newfoundland)

Preparation: 20 minutes
Cook: 25 to 30 minutes
Makes 20 cups (5 L) or 40 servings

Calories per half-cup (125 mL) serving: 241
Grams of protein per serving: 7.1
Grams of fat per serving: 14.3
Grams of carbohydrate per serving: 24.3
Grams of fibre per serving: 3.4

STRAWBERRY PURÉE

2 cups	fresh strawberries	500 mL
	or	
1	package (300 g)	1
	frozen unsweetened strawberries	
	Sugar (optional)	

Wash strawberries, remove hulls; cook gently on low heat until softened; cool. If berries are frozen, allow them to thaw. Purée fresh or frozen strawberries in food processor or blender until smooth. Taste and add sugar, if necessary. Serve sauce warm over pancakes.

Makes approximately 1 cup (250 mL)

Preparation: 10 minutes
Cook: 4 to 5 minutes
Makes 8 pancakes and 8 servings
Calories per serving of pancake with purée: 170
Grams of protein per serving: 4.7
Grams of fat per serving: 6.8
Grams of carbohydrate per serving: 24.4
Grams of fibre per serving: 3.4

WHOLE WHEAT PANCAKES WITH STRAWBERRY PURÉE

Caroline Beaurivage, Abbotsford, British Columbia

Whole wheat pancakes that are light textured like these will become a treasured recipe. Serve with sliced fresh fruit or the Strawberry Purée for a good start to your day.

1⅓ cups	whole wheat flour	325 mL
3 tbsp.	brown sugar	45 mL
1 tbsp.	baking powder	15 mL
1 tsp.	cinnamon	5 mL
¼ tsp.	salt	1 mL
1¼ cups	2 percent milk	300 mL
1	egg, beaten	1
3 tbsp.	vegetable oil	45 mL
½ tsp.	vanilla extract	2 mL
	Oil (optional)	

Mix flour, sugar, baking powder, cinnamon, and salt.

In separate bowl, beat together milk, egg, oil, and vanilla extract. Add liquid ingredients to dry, mixing until almost smooth (disregard small lumps).

Heat skillet or griddle over medium heat; brush with oil (optional for non-stick pans). For each pancake, pour ¼ cup (50 mL) batter into skillet. When underside is brown and bubbles break on topside (after 1½ to 2 minutes), flip over and cook 30 to 60 seconds, or until second side is golden brown. Serve hot.

Variation: Fresh or frozen unsweetened raspberries or blueberries or fresh peaches could replace strawberries.

MENU SUGGESTION

Traditional breakfast dishes are often high in fat. Here's a lower-fat, higher-fibre version of an old favourite. Serve with honey-sweetened plain yoghurt and fresh fruit slices. (Laura Sevenhuysen, R.D., Winnipeg, Manitoba)

Preparation: 5 minutes
Cook: 3 to 5 minutes
Makes 6 servings

Calories per serving: 80
Grams of protein per serving: 4.9
Grams of fat per serving: 0.7
Grams of carbohydrate per serving: 14.3
Grams of fibre per serving: 2.1

FRENCH TOAST
Lise Parisien, Cornwall, Ontario.

Serve this low-fat breakfast bread with honey or maple syrup, sweetened plain yoghurt, fresh fruit, and wheat germ or Granola (page 180).

4	egg whites	4
2 tbsp.	skim milk	25 mL
½ tsp.	vanilla extract	2 mL
Pinch	nutmeg, cinnamon	Pinch
6	slices whole wheat bread	6

Beat together egg whites, milk, vanilla, and nutmeg until frothy. Pour into large flat dish; dip both sides of bread into mixture.

In large non-stick or lightly buttered skillet, cook bread until brown on one side. Flip and cook other side. Serve immediately.

For one serving: Place ⅓ cup (75 mL) of oat mixture into a deep bowl. Add ¾ cup (175 mL) water and a dash of salt. Microwave on High (100 percent) for 2 minutes; stir. Microwave 1 to 2 minutes longer or cook in small saucepan on top of stove for about 5 minutes.

Preparation: 5 minutes
Microwave: 3 to 4 minutes
Makes 2½ cups (625 mL) or 7 servings

Calories per serving: 143
Grams of protein per serving: 5.8
Grams of fat per serving: 1.6
Grams of carbohydrate per serving: 26.8
Grams of fibre per serving: 3.9

NOT YOUR SAME OLD OATS
Michael G. Baylis, Toronto, Ontario

This breakfast cereal combines the goodness of oats and oat bran with high-fibre grains like cracked wheat. The texture can be varied by altering the proportion of grains. Serve with milk and sliced fresh fruit if desired.

1 cup	large-flake rolled oats	250 mL
⅔ cup	five-grain cereal	150 mL
½ cup	oat bran	125 mL
⅓ cup	medium bulgur (cracked wheat)	75 mL

In large bowl, combine oats, cereal, oat bran, and bulgur. Store in tightly closed container.

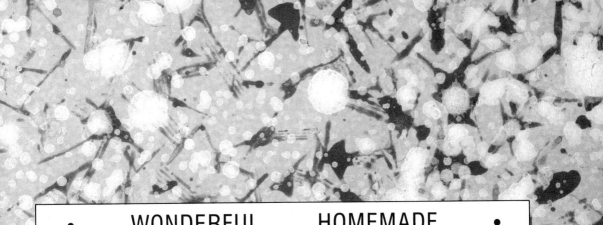

BAKED GOODS

Not all baked goods are created equal. Today's nutrition-conscious consumers are seeking recipes that will increase the complex carbohydrates and fibre in their diet.

Breads and other baked goods made with whole wheat flour have a delicious nutty flavour and are a healthier choice than those made with all-purpose flour. However, a word of caution: you may replace only up to 50 percent of all-purpose with whole wheat flour in old favourite recipes without adjusting the recipe. Whole wheat as well as rye flours produce heavier baked items than all-purpose flour does. Thus, the addition of some all-purpose flour will improve volume and texture of baked items.

Types of Flour

All-Purpose: as the name implies, this white flour is of general use but is especially suitable for yeast breads, tea biscuits, muffins, and quick breads.

Cake and pastry flour: by replacing all-purpose flour with cake and pastry, you can reduce the sugar and fat in a cake recipe. Cake flour has a lower protein content than other flours, which contributes to a more delicate crumb. It also has less gluten, so it tenderizes with less shortening. (To replace all-purpose flour with cake and pastry flour: 1 cup (250 mL) all-purpose flour = 1 cup (250 mL) plus 2 tbsp. (25 mL) cake and pastry flour.)

Whole wheat: this brown flour contains bran that has been reduced to fine particles.

Rye flour: the cereal grain rye is milled into a flour with a characteristic dark colour and strong flavour. Generally, it is used in breads, but it may be added to cookies or muffins.

Graham flour: you can use graham flour as you do whole wheat flour. The bran particles added to this flour are larger than those in whole wheat flour.

Oat Bran: you certainly do not need a recipe to incorporate oat bran into your baking. Oat bran can be added in small quantities as a replacement for flour. Just don't use too much, or the finished food will be gummy and heavy.

FREEZING TIPS

Wrap baked goods (after thorough cooling) in airtight plastic bags or a double thickness of aluminum foil. Generally, thaw in original freezer wrapper at room temperature. Thaw baked goods only in the amounts needed as they soon stale. To freshen breads, rolls, muffins, or biscuits that have been frozen, then thawed at room temperature, wrap in foil and heat in 300°F (160°C) oven for 5 to 15 minutes.

FREEZER STORAGE

Cookies: 12 months

Quick Breads and Muffins: 4 to 5 months

Yeast Breads: 3 months

Cake: 5 to 6 months for plain; 3 months for iced

Pies: 3 months

WHEAT GERM AS A REPLACEMENT FOR NUTS

Wheat germ can replace nuts as a garnish on cookies, muffins, cakes, salads, vegetables, and casseroles.

In order to develop a crispier, toasted texture in wheat germ, roast in a moderate oven (about 350°F/180°C) for 10 to 15 minutes, or in a non-stick skillet over medium heat, stirring frequently.

Herbs, spices, or cheese may be added to wheat germ for sprinkling on soups, casseroles, vegetables, and salads.

Measuring Tips

Let's take a minute to talk about proper measuring, since nowhere is this more critical than with baked goods. Since Imperial as well as metric measures are used in Canada, be sure to use only one system for a recipe; do not combine them. Always use standard measuring utensils for both dry and liquid ingredients.

LIQUID MEASURES (*glass, Pyrex, or plastic with a lip*) come in:
Imperial: 1-cup, 2-cup, and 4-cup sizes
Metric: 250 mL, 500 mL, and 1 L sizes
  Place cup on level surface and fill to the required amount; check at eye level.

DRY MEASURES (*usually stackable cups of varying sizes*) come in graduated sizes:
Imperial: ¼-cup, ⅓-cup, ½-cup, and 1-cup sizes
Metric − 50 mL, 125 mL, and 250 mL sizes
  Fill to overflowing with dry ingredient; level off with a straight-edged knife or metal spatula; do not pack down.

SMALL MEASURES OR SPOONS come in:
Imperial: ¼-teaspoon, ½-teaspoon, 1-teaspoon, and 1-tablespoon sizes
Metric: 1 mL, 2 mL, 5 mL, 15 mL, and 25 mL sizes
  Use these to measure small quantities of both dry and liquid ingredients. Level small dry measures in similar fashion as large dry measures.

Photos: Carrot Bran Muffins, page 191 (facing page); Grandma's Unsweetened Rolled Oat Cookies, page 194 (overleaf)

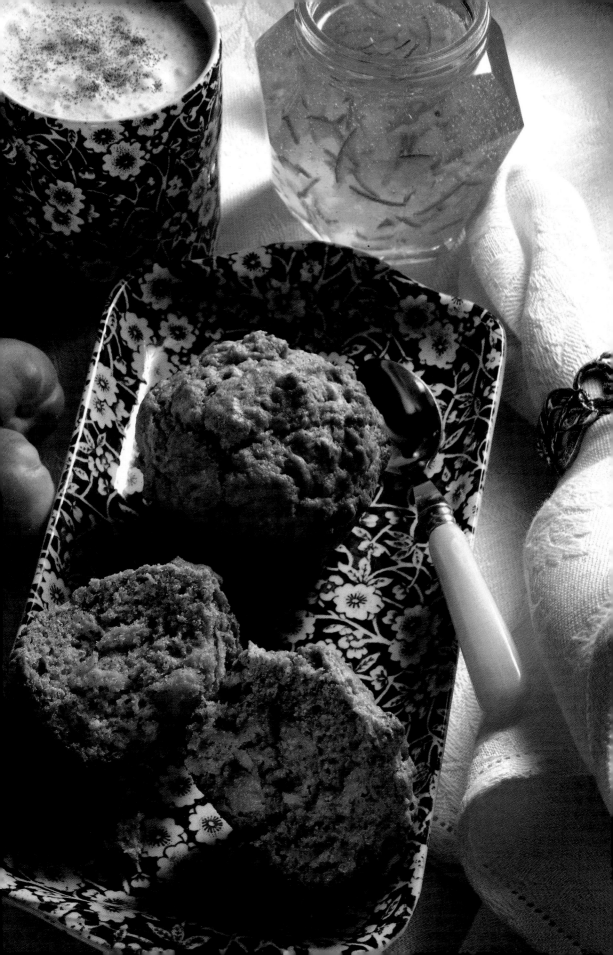

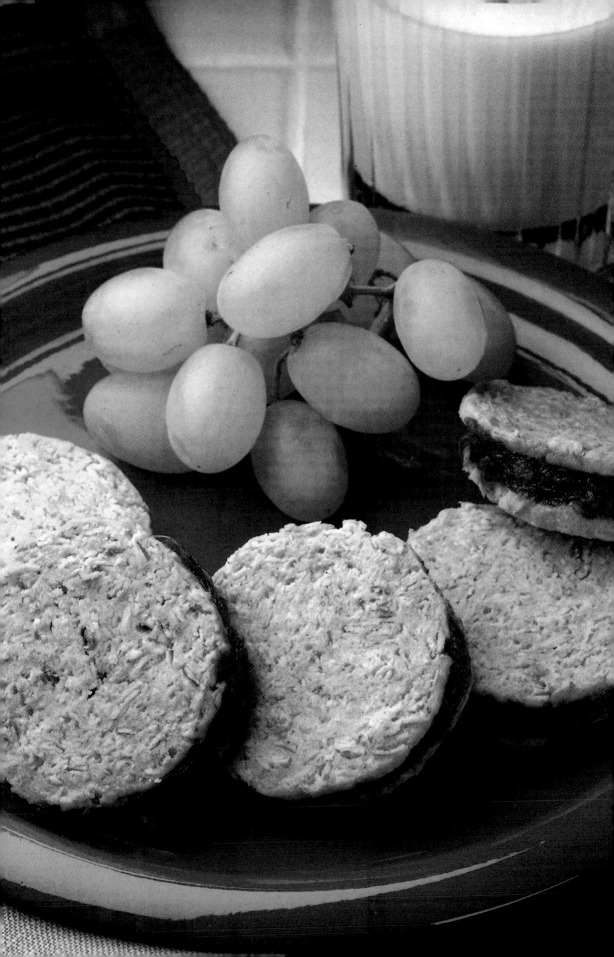

APPLE SAUCE SNACK CAKES
Elaine Durst, Westbank, British Columbia

These muffin-like cakes are a treat for kid's lunch boxes or for breakfast. For extra fibre, slide a wedge of unpeeled apple into the top of each snack cake before baking.

½ cup	butter or margarine	125 mL
1½ cups	granulated sugar	375 mL
2	eggs	2
1 tsp.	vanilla extract	5 mL
2 cups	all-purpose flour	500 mL
1 tbsp.	baking powder	15 mL
1 tsp.	baking soda	5 mL
1½ tsp.	ground cinnamon	7 mL
1 tsp.	ground allspice	5 mL
½ tsp.	ground cloves	2 mL
2 cups	unsweetened apple sauce	500 mL

In large bowl, cream butter and sugar. Beat in eggs and vanilla until light and fluffy.

Sift together flour, baking powder, baking soda, and spices. Add to creamed mixture alternately with apple sauce, mixing well after each addition.

Spoon into paper-lined muffin cups, filling each about two-thirds full. Bake in 400°F (200°C) oven for about 20 minutes, or until firm to the touch.

Preparation: 15 minutes
Cook: about 20 minutes
Makes 16 medium cupcakes

Calories per cupcake: 200
Grams of protein per cupcake: 2.5
Grams of fat per cupcake: 6.4
Grams of carbohydrate per cupcake: 33.8
Grams of fibre per cupcake: 1.0

DILLY BREAD
Carla Murphy, North Bay, Ontario

Cottage cheese adds extra nutrients to this casserole bread. Enjoy with Manitoba Vegetable Soup (page 62).

1 tsp.	granulated sugar	5 mL
¼ cup	warm water	50 mL
1	package active dry yeast	1
1 cup	low-fat (2 percent) cottage cheese	250 mL
1 tbsp.	grated onion	15 mL
2 tbsp.	granulated sugar	25 mL
1 tbsp.	dill seed	15 mL
1 tsp.	salt	5 mL
¼ tsp.	baking soda	1 mL
1 tbsp.	butter or margarine, melted	15 mL
1	egg, beaten	1
2¾ cups	all-purpose flour	675 mL

In bowl, dissolve sugar in warm water. Sprinkle yeast over and let stand 10 minutes, or until foamy.

In large bowl, combine yeast mixture, cottage cheese, onion, sugar, dill seed, salt, baking soda, butter, and egg. Gradually stir in flour until smooth (this will be a stiff dough). Turn out on lightly floured surface and knead until smooth and elastic.

Place dough in lightly greased 8-inch (1.2 L) round casserole, turning to grease all over. Cover bowl loosely and let stand in warm place about 1½ hours, or until doubled in volume. Bake in 350°F (180°C) oven for about 45 minutes. (Do not underbake, a crisp crust is desirable.)

MENU SUGGESTION

For a meal with a northern flair, serve baked Arctic char with wild rice, tossed salad with Lemon Pesto Dressing (page 155), and this delicious Dilly Bread with its unique flavour and low fat content. Cranberry crisp is a delightful finish to the meal. (Elsie De Roose, R.Dt., Yellowknife, Northwest Territories)

Preparation: 2 hours
Cook: 45 to 50 minutes
Makes 1 round loaf or about 12 slices

Calories per slice: 148
Grams of protein per slice: 6.3
Grams of fat per slice: 2.1
Grams of carbohydrate per slice: 25.4
Grams of fibre per slice: 0.9

WHOLE WHEAT PIZZA DOUGH
Melanie Galvin, Thunder Bay, Ontario.

Whole wheat flour and herbs provide a tasty pizza crust to use with your own favourite topping combinations or for Chicken Pizza (page 74). Herbs and garlic may be omitted when a plainer crust is required. Melanie Galvin tells us she frequently prepared pizza for her roommates while she was at university.

1¼ cups	all-purpose flour	375 mL
1¼ cups	whole wheat flour	375 mL
1	package quick-rise instant yeast	1
1 tsp.	granulated sugar	5 mL
½ tsp.	salt	2 mL
½ tsp.	dried basil	2 mL
½ tsp.	dried oregano	2 mL
¼ tsp.	garlic powder	1 mL
½ cup	water	125 mL
¼ cup	2 percent milk	50 mL
3 tbsp.	olive oil	45 mL

Combine flours, yeast, sugar, salt, and seasonings.

In small saucepan on low heat, heat water, milk, and olive oil until hot to touch (125°F/50°C). Stir into dry ingredients. Knead on floured surface until smooth and elastic. Cover and let rest for 10 minutes.

Cut dough in half; roll each half into 12-inch (30 cm) round. Place each on non-stick or lightly greased baking or pizza pan. Flute edge to form shell to hold fillings. Cover; let rise in warm place for about 30 minutes.

Add toppings; bake in 425°F (220°C) oven on bottom rack for about 15 minutes.

Variation: Replace ½ cup (125 mL) whole wheat flour with ½ cup (125 mL) oat bran.

Preparation: 20 minutes
Cook: 15 minutes
Makes 2 pizza shells

Calories per serving (1/6 shell): 122
Grams of protein per serving: 3.4
Grams of fat per serving: 3.7
Grams of carbohydrate per serving: 19.4
Grams of fibre per serving: 2.0

SPEEDY YAM 'N' EGG ROLLS

Linda Terra, Calgary, Alberta

These soft and golden fruit buns are tasty and nutritious. Serve warm for breakfast or at tea-time. If you use canned yams for this recipe, reserve the liquid. If you cook and mash yams, use the cooking liquid.

3 cups	all-purpose flour, divided	750 mL
1½ cups	whole wheat flour	375 mL
½ cup	oat bran	125 mL
¼ cup	skim-milk powder	50 mL
2 tbsp.	grated orange rind	25 mL
½ tsp.	salt	2 mL
¾ cup	currants, washed and dried	175 mL
1	package quick-rise instant yeast	1
¾ cup	cooked mashed yams, reserve liquid	175 mL
¼ cup	butter or margarine, melted	50 mL
¼ cup	liquid honey	50 mL
1 cup	yam liquid	250 mL
2	eggs, slightly beaten	2
	Melted butter	

In large bowl, mix 2 cups (500 mL) all-purpose flour, whole wheat flour, oat bran, skim-milk powder, orange rind, salt, currants, and yeast.

In small saucepan on low heat, heat yams, butter, honey, and yam liquid until hot to touch (125°F/50°C). Stir hot mixture and eggs into dry ingredients.

Stir in enough remaining flour to make a soft dough. Turn out on lightly floured surface and knead until smooth and elastic. Cover and let rest 10 minutes.

With sharp knife, cut dough into 16 equal pieces; shape each into smooth ball, tucking ends under. Place seam side down on non-stick or lightly greased baking sheet about 2 inches (5 cm) apart. Cover and let rise until doubled in bulk, about 1 hour.

Bake in 375°F (190°C) oven for about 15 minutes, or until golden brown. For shiny tops, brush baked buns with melted butter while still hot.

MENU SUGGESTION

These rolls are a welcome change from the usual breakfast fare and the oat bran and yams contribute complex carbohydrates and fibre. For a breakfast that provides protein and calcium as well, serve these rolls with cantaloupe melon baskets with cottage cheese. (Roxanne Eyer, R.D., Winnipeg, Manitoba)

Preparation: 2½ hours
Cook: 15 to 20 minutes
Makes 16 rolls

Calories per roll: 220
Grams of protein per roll: 6.2
Grams of fat per roll: 4.2
Grams of carbohydrate per roll: 40.5
Grams of fibre per roll: 2.8

SUPER HEALTH BREAD
Alma R. Price, Toronto, Ontario

This nutrition-packed bread was a runner-up in the baked goods category. It tastes great served with milk, juice, or coffee.

½ cup	boiling water	125 mL
1 cup	raisins	250 mL
1	egg, beaten	1
1 cup	lightly packed brown sugar	250 mL
1 cup	buttermilk	250 mL
1 cup	whole wheat flour	250 mL
1 cup	rolled oats	250 mL
1 cup	high-fibre bran cereal	250 mL
¼ cup	wheat germ	50 mL
1 ½ tsp.	baking soda	7 mL
½ tsp.	salt	2 mL

Pour boiling water over raisins; allow to cool. Stir in egg, sugar, and buttermilk.

In medium bowl, combine flour, oats, cereal, wheat germ, baking soda, and salt. Stir in egg mixture until thoroughly combined. Pour into 9 × 5-inch (2 L) non-stick or lightly greased loaf pan. Bake in 350°F (180°C) oven for about 45 minutes or until tester inserted in centre comes out clean. Allow to cool before removing from pan.

MENU SUGGESTION
This bread is a healthy accompaniment to almost any meal. Serve it with Spicy Potato Soup (page 65), citrus salad, and Strawberry Yoghurt Pie (page 218). (Jean Norman, R.Dt., St. John's, Newfoundland)

Preparation: 15 minutes
Cook: 45 minutes
Makes 1 loaf of about 16 slices

Calories per slice: 151
Grams of protein per slice: 4.0
Grams of fat per slice: 1.3
Grams of carbohydrate per slice: 34.3
Grams of fibre per slice: 3.7

WHOLE WHEAT BISCUITS
Karen Dewar, Teulon, Manitoba

These tasty biscuits are perfect with soup or a salad.

2 cups	whole wheat flour	500 mL
1 tbsp.	baking powder	15 mL
1 tbsp.	parsley flakes	15 mL
⅓ cup	butter or margarine	75 mL
¾ cup	2 percent milk	175 mL
1	egg, slightly beaten	1

MENU SUGGESTION

These whole wheat biscuits are great fresh from the oven and are an excellent accompaniment to soups or stews. Serve with Beef Barley Soup (page 71), crunchy and colourful raw vegetables, an apple, and a glass of low-fat milk for a filling schoolday lunch or for a warming supper after a day on the ski trails. (Penny Lobdell, R.D.N., Kelowna, British Columbia)

In medium bowl, combine flour, baking powder, and parsley flakes. Cut in butter until mixture resembles fine crumbs.

Combine milk and egg; add to dry ingredients, stirring with fork to make a soft dough.

Turn out onto lightly floured surface and knead about 10 times. Roll to ½-inch (1 cm) thickness. Cut with floured 2-inch (5 cm) round cookie cutter. Place on baking pan; bake in 450°F (220°C) oven for 10 to 12 minutes, or until golden.

Preparation: 15 minutes
Cook: 10 to 12 minutes
Makes 1½ dozen biscuits

Calories per biscuit: 82
Grams of protein per biscuit: 2.4
Grams of fat per biscuit: 4.0
Grams of carbohydrate per biscuit: 9.9
Grams of fibre per biscuit: 1.6

Carrots and zucchini are great in cakes and muffins but have you tried beets? Cook whole beets until tender then puree them, skin and all, in your blender or food processor. Substitute beet puree or grated raw beets in your recipes calling for pureed or grated carrots or zucchini. The beets will provide a dark, rich colour.

CARROT BRAN MUFFINS
Steve Holodinsky, Simcoe, Ontario

Two favourites, carrot and bran, are combined in this tasty muffin. A great snack or start to your day.

1¼ cups	whole wheat flour	300 mL
1¼ cups	high-fibre bran cereal	300 mL
1 tsp.	baking powder	5 mL
1 tsp.	baking soda	5 mL
1 tsp.	ground cinnamon	5 mL
½ tsp.	ground nutmeg	2 mL
½ tsp.	salt	2 mL
2	eggs	2
1 cup	grated carrots	250 mL
¾ cup	buttermilk	175 mL
⅓ cup	firmly packed brown sugar	75 mL
¼ cup	vegetable oil	50 mL
½ cup	raisins	125 mL

In large bowl, combine flour, cereal, baking powder, baking soda, and spices.

In separate bowl, beat eggs thoroughly; blend carrots, buttermilk, brown sugar, and vegetable oil. Add to dry ingredients, stirring just until moistened. Stir in raisins.

Spoon batter into muffin tins lined with paper baking cups, filling about three-quarters full. Bake in 400°F (200°C) oven for 20 minutes, or until tops of muffins spring back when lightly touched.

MENU SUGGESTION
Start your day off right with one of these muffins for fibre and a Berry Shake (page 239) for calcium and vitamins. (Helen Haresign, R.P.Dt., Toronto, Ontario)

Preparation: 15 minutes
Cook: 20 minutes
Makes 12 muffins

Calories per muffin: 166
Grams of protein per muffin: 4.4
Grams of fat per muffin: 5.9
Grams of carbohydrate per muffin: 27.8
Grams of fibre per muffin: 4.6

GIB'S GOURMET MUFFINS
Gilbert H. Ducharme, Ottawa, Ontario

Gib's bran muffins replace eggs with egg whites, sugar with honey and molasses. Raisins and unsweetened pineapple make this a moist and fruity muffin that freezes well.

1½ cups	whole wheat flour	375 mL
2 cups	natural wheat bran	500 mL
1½ tsp.	baking powder	7 mL
¼ tsp.	baking soda	1 mL
¼ tsp.	ground nutmeg	1 mL
¼ tsp.	ground cinnamon	1 mL
1 cup	skim milk	250 mL
2	egg whites, lightly beaten	2
½ cup	safflower oil	125 mL
½ cup	liquid honey	125 mL
½ cup	molasses	125 mL
2 cups	raisins	500 mL
1 cup	crushed unsweetened pineapple, well drained	250 mL

In large bowl, combine flour, bran, baking powder, baking soda, and spices.

In another bowl, combine milk, egg whites, oil, honey, and molasses. Stir in raisins and pineapple. Add to dry ingredients, stirring just until moistened; do not overmix. Spoon into lightly greased or paper-lined muffin cups, filling three-quarters full. Bake in 350°F (180°C) oven for about 20 to 25 minutes, or until tops of muffins spring back when lightly touched.

MENU SUGGESTION

Since these moist and tasty fibre-packed muffins have more sugar and fat than some of the other bread or muffin recipes, complement them with a meal that's lower in calories: tomato juice, vegetable chicken salad with low-fat dressing, and low-fat yoghurt with fresh berries and cinnamon. (Carol Carter, R.D.N., Victoria, British Columbia)

Preparation: 15 minutes
Cook: 20 to 25 minutes
Makes 16 muffins

Calories per muffin: 243
Grams of protein per muffin: 4.1
Grams of fat per muffin: 7.2
Grams of carbohydrate per muffin: 46.1
Grams of fibre per muffin: 5.1

CRANBERRY OAT MUFFINS
Laura M. Hawthorn, Bracebridge, Ontario

This tart, tasty muffin can be enjoyed year-round if you freeze cranberries when they are available fresh in the fall. If you live in the Muskoka region of Ontario as Laura Hawthorn does, you will be able to obtain fresh cranberries in season locally. It is unnecessary to thaw cranberries before using in this recipe.

¾ cup	rolled oats	175 mL
1½ cups	all-purpose flour, divided	375 mL
1 cup	granulated sugar	250 mL
2 tsp.	baking powder	10 mL
½ tsp.	salt	2 mL
½ cup	butter or margarine	125 mL
1½ cups	fresh or frozen cranberries, chopped	375 mL
2 tsp.	grated lemon rind	10 mL
⅔ cup	2 percent milk	150 mL
1	egg, beaten	1

TOPPING

4 tsp.	ground cinnamon	20 mL
2 tsp.	granulated sugar	10 mL

In food processor or blender, process oats until very fine. Combine oats, flour (except for 2 tbsp./25 mL), sugar, baking powder, and salt. Cut in butter with a pastry blender or food processor until mixture resembles coarse crumbs.

Toss cranberries with reserved flour; stir into flour mixture.

Combine lemon rind, milk, and egg; mix thoroughly. Add to dry ingredients, stirring just until moistened; do not overmix. Spoon into lightly greased or paper-lined muffin cups, filling three-quarters full.

Combine cinnamon and sugar; sprinkle over muffins. Bake in 400°F (200°C) oven for 20 to 25 minutes, or until tops of muffins spring back when lightly touched.

MENU SUGGESTION

These tangy muffins, along with a fresh fruit medley, low-fat cottage cheese, and 2 percent milk, make a great get-up-and-go breakfast that contributes fibre and keeps fat under control. (Rosemarie Russel, R.P.Dt., London, Ontario)

Preparation: 15 minutes
Cook: 20 to 25 minutes
Makes 12 medium muffins.

Calories per muffin: 227
Grams of protein per muffin: 3.5
Grams of fat per muffin: 8.6
Grams of carbohydrate per muffin: 34.8
Grams of fibre per serving: 1.4

GRANDMA'S UNSWEETENED ROLLED OAT COOKIES

Grace Jackson, Winnipeg, Manitoba

This recipe is aptly named: it is as warm and comforting as when grandma made it. The unsweetened cookie tastes like a Scottish oat cake; the sweeter date filling compliments the oatmeal.

COOKIE

1½ cups	all-purpose flour	375 mL
1½ cups	rolled oats	375 mL
1 tsp.	baking soda	5 mL
½ cup	shortening	125 mL
½ cup	hot water	125 mL

FILLING

2 cups	chopped dates	500 mL
½ cup	water	125 mL
¼ cup	granulated sugar	50 mL
1 tsp.	vanilla extract	5 mL

Combine flour, oats, and baking soda. Cut in shortening until mixture resembles coarse crumbs. Add sufficient water to shape dough into a roll. Wrap in waxed paper; refrigerate overnight.

Cut cookie dough into thin wafers (⅛ inch/3 mm). Place on non-stick or lightly greased cookie sheet. Bake in 325°F (160°C) oven for about 10 minutes.

To prepare filling, cook dates, water, and sugar on low heat for about 30 minutes; stir occasionally. Stir in vanilla.

When cookies and filling are cool, spread about 1 tbsp. (15 mL) date filling between two cookies.

Preparation: overnight
Cook: 30 minutes
Makes 3 dozen filled cookies

Calories per cookie: 88
Grams of protein per cookie: 1.3
Grams of fat per cookie: 3.0
Grams of carbohydrate per cookie: 14.7
Grams of fibre per cookie: 1.2

SUNFLOWER COOKIES
Alexa Miller, Dartmouth, Nova Scotia

The crunchiness of nuts and seeds and the sweetness of raisins and chocolate chips makes this healthy cookie one that the young and the not-so-young will enjoy.

½ cup	butter or margarine	125 mL
¾ cup	lightly packed brown sugar	175 mL
¾ cup	granulated sugar	175 mL
1	egg, beaten	1
½ tsp.	vanilla extract	2 mL
½ tsp.	baking soda	2 mL
2 tsp.	hot water	10 mL
1 cup	unsalted shelled sunflower seeds	250 mL
½ cup	all-purpose flour	125 mL
½ cup	whole wheat flour	125 mL
½ cup	large-flake rolled oats	125 mL
½ cup	chocolate chips	125 mL
½ cup	raisins	125 mL
⅓ cup	natural wheat bran	75 mL
⅓ cup	wheat germ	75 mL
1 tsp.	salt	5 mL

Preparation: 15 minutes
Cook: 10 minutes
Makes 5 dozen cookies

Calories per cookie: 69
Grams of protein per cookie: 1.3
Grams of fat per cookie: 3.3
Grams of carbohydrate per cookie: 9.5
Grams of fibre per cookie: 0.7

In large bowl, cream butter, brown sugar, and granulated sugar until fluffy. Stir in egg, vanilla, and baking soda dissolved in hot water. Add sunflower seeds, flours, oats, chocolate chips, raisins, bran, wheat germ, and salt; combine thoroughly.

Drop batter a spoonful at a time onto non-stick or lightly greased cookie sheets. Bake in 350°F (180°C) oven for about 10 minutes.

MATRIMONIAL CAKE
Margaret Haresign, Winnipeg, Manitoba.

One of the young men who tasted this cake was overheard to say,
"This cake is a close rival to my mother's recipe."

1½ cups	all-purpose flour	375 mL
1½ cups	rolled oats	375 mL
1 cup	lightly packed brown sugar	250 mL
1 tsp.	baking soda	5 mL
1 cup	butter or margarine	250 mL

DATE FILLING

1 lb.	dates, chopped (about 4 cups/1 L)	500 g
1½ cups	water	375 mL
2 tbsp.	lemon juice	25 mL

In large bowl, combine flour, oats, brown sugar, and baking soda. Cut in butter with pastry blender or in food processor until mixture is crumbly. Press half the crumb mixture into non-stick or lightly greased 9 × 13-inch (3.5 L) baking pan.

To make date filling: In covered saucepan over low heat, cook dates and water until thickened and smooth, about 15 minutes; stir occasionally. (You may need to add extra water while cooking if mixture becomes too thick.) Stir in lemon juice. Spread over crumb layer; sprinkle with remaining crumb mixture. Bake in 350°F (180°C) oven for about 35 minutes, or until lightly brown. Cut into bars.

Preparation: 20 minutes
Cook: about 35 minutes
Makes 42 bars

Calories per bar: 113
Grams of protein per bar: 1.2
Grams of fat per bar: 4.5
Grams of carbohydrate per bar: 18.1
Grams of fibre per bar: 1.2

HARVEST RAISIN CAKE
Maryanne Cattrysse, Simcoe, Ontario

We prepared this moist and spice-filled cake in a large oblong pan. However, it could be baked in a tube pan. We have also baked the batter as muffins.

1½ cups	granulated sugar	375 mL
1 cup	whole wheat flour	250 mL
1 cup	all-purpose flour	250 mL
2 tsp.	baking powder	10 mL
1 tsp.	baking soda	5 mL
½ tsp.	salt	2 mL
1½ tsp.	ground cinnamon	7 mL
¼ tsp.	ground cloves	1 mL
¼ tsp.	ground nutmeg	1 mL
¼ tsp.	ground ginger	1 mL
4	eggs	4
1	can (14 oz./398 mL) pumpkin	1
½ cup	vegetable oil	125 mL
1 cup	high-fibre bran cereal	250 mL
1 cup	raisins	250 mL

In large bowl, combine sugar, flours, baking powder, baking soda, salt, and spices.

In second bowl, beat eggs, pumpkin, oil, and cereal. Add flour mixture, mixing only until combined. Stir in raisins. Spread evenly in non-stick or lightly greased 9 × 13-inch (3.5 L) pan. Bake in 350°F (180°C) oven for about 40 minutes, or until tester inserted in centre comes out clean. Cool completely on wire rack.

Variations
Tube pan: Bake in 350°F (180°C) oven for about 50 minutes.
Muffins: Bake in 350°F (180°C) for about 20 minutes.

MENU SUGGESTION

This cake provides a variety of types of fibre all in one recipe. For even more fibre, serve it after a meal of French-Canadian pea soup and cottage cheese with fresh fruit. This menu includes foods from all four food groups. (Ellen Vogel, R.D., Winnipeg, Manitoba)

Preparation: 20 minutes
Cook: about 40 minutes
Makes: 24 to 30 pieces in 9 × 13-inch (3.5 L) pan, 20 slices in 10-inch (25 cm) tube pan, or about 3 dozen muffins.

Calories per serving of cake: 135
Grams of protein per serving: 2.4
Grams of fat per serving: 4.5
Grams of carbohydrate per serving: 23.1
Grams of fibre per serving: 1.8

FRUIT SQUARES
Joanne Hoyle, Toronto, Ontario

Pack these spicy fruit squares as a healthy treat for the brown-bagger, or as a treat after school with a glass of milk.

In recipes using a whole egg, you can often substitute either one or two egg whites. If a recipe calls for two eggs, use one whole egg and two egg whites, for example in meatloaf, hamburgers, pancakes, quickbreads, muffins, or salad dressing. If a recipe calls for two egg yolks, use one whole egg instead. This substitution will decrease the fat and cholesterol content of the recipe.

2 cups	finely diced unpeeled apples	500 mL
½ cup	raisins	125 mL
½ cup	chopped dates	125 mL
2	eggs, beaten	2
¾ cup	lightly packed brown sugar	175 mL
½ cup	vegetable oil	125 mL
1 tsp.	vanilla extract	5 mL
1 cup	all-purpose flour	250 mL
1 tsp.	baking soda	5 mL
1 tsp.	ground cinnamon	5 mL

In medium bowl, combine apples, raisins, and dates. In large bowl, combine eggs, sugar, oil, and vanilla.

In a third bowl, combine flour, baking soda, and cinnamon; add to egg mixture. Stir in fruit. Spread in nonstick or lightly greased 9 × 13-inch (3.5 L) baking pan. Bake in 350°F (180°C) oven for about 25 minutes, or until tester inserted in centre comes out clean.

Preparation: 15 minutes
Cook: about 25 minutes
Makes 20 to 25 squares

Calories per square: 110
Grams of protein per square: 1.2
Grams of fat per square: 4.7
Grams of carbohydrate per square: 16.4
Grams of fibre per square: 0.8

HEALTHY CHEESE 'N' HERB BREAD
Margaret Howard, Toronto, Ontario

"This is a bread my family enjoys and I have served for many years as an accompaniment to brunch or a salad supper," writes *Margaret Howard.*

2 cups	all-purpose flour	500 mL
1 cup	whole wheat flour	250 mL
½ cup	rolled oats	125 mL
1 tbsp.	granulated sugar	15 mL
2 tsp.	baking powder	10 mL
½ tsp.	baking soda	2 mL
1 tsp.	dried basil	5 mL
½ tsp.	dried oregano	2 mL
½ tsp.	salt	2 mL
¼ cup	cold butter or margarine	50 mL
1 cup	shredded Swiss cheese	250 mL
1	egg	1
1 cup	buttermilk	250 mL
2 tbsp.	sesame seeds	25 mL

Preparation: 10 minutes
Cook: 25 to 30 minutes
Makes 8 to 10 servings

Calories per serving: 259
Grams of protein per serving: 9.9
Grams of fat per serving: 9.9
Grams of carbohydrate per serving: 33.2
Grams of fibre per serving: 2.5

In medium bowl, combine flours, oats, sugar, baking powder, baking soda, herbs, and salt. Cut in butter with a pastry blender until mixture resembles fine crumbs. Stir in cheese.

Beat together egg and buttermilk; add to dry ingredients, stirring with fork to make a soft moist dough. Turn batter into 8-inch (1.2 L) round non-stick or lightly greased pan. Sprinkle with sesame seeds. Bake in 400°F (200°C) oven for 25-30 minutes, or until tester inserted in centre comes out clean. Cut into wedges to serve.

HOMEMADE BAGELS
Monique Clément, Gloucester, Ontario

Monique Clément wrote, "Bagels are as varied as the imagination will allow—onion, sesame seed, poppyseed, white, rye, salted, plain, whole wheat, cinnamon, raisin, and on and on." She added, "It doesn't take as long to do as it looks and is very rewarding to taste!" Serve these as a breakfast treat—split and toasted, spread with peanut butter, butter or margarine, honey or jam.

GLAZE (optional)

1	egg white, lightly beaten	1
1 tbsp.	water	15 mL

3 tbsp.	liquid honey or granulated sugar	45 mL
1½ cups	warm water	375 mL
2	packages active dry yeast	2
2 cups	all-purpose flour	500 mL
1 cup	whole wheat flour	250 mL
½ cup	oat bran	125 mL
1 tbsp.	salt	15 mL
2 quarts	water	2 L
1 tbsp.	granulated sugar	15 mL
1 tsp.	cornmeal	5 mL

Toppings: sesame seeds, poppy seeds, garlic powder

MENU SUGGESTION

No more soggy sandwiches! These bagels contain a variety of types of fibre and are ideal for the lunch box. Fill them with tuna salad and add celery sticks, tomato wedges, and a thermos of milk for a satisfying lunch. (Laura Sevenhuysen, R.D., Winnipeg, Manitoba)

In large bowl, dissolve honey in warm water. Sprinkle yeast over and let stand 10 minutes, or until foamy.

To dissolved yeast, mixing well between each addition, stir in flours, oat bran, and salt. (Add extra flour, if necessary, to obtain a dough that is solid when pinched with fingers.) Turn out onto lightly floured surface and knead for 8 minutes, or until smooth and elastic.

Place dough in lightly greased bowl, turning to grease all over. Cover bowl tightly with plastic wrap and then with a tea towel; place in cool oven with a large bowl of steaming water for about one hour, or until doubled in volume.

You can make bagel crackers from any leftover stale bagels. Slice bagels into thin circles. Place on a baking sheet that has been lightly greased. Bake in 300°F (150°C) oven for about 25 minutes, or until crisp. Cool on rack.

Preparation: 2 hours
Cook: 20 to 25 minutes
Makes 10 bagels

Calories per bagel: 170
Grams of protein per bagel: 5.6
Grams of fat per bagel: 0.9
Grams of carbohydrate per bagel: 35.7
Grams of fibre per bagel: 3.0

Turn dough out onto lightly floured surface and punch down. With sharp knife, cut into 10 equal pieces; shape each into smooth ball. Allow to relax for about 4 minutes; flatten with palm of hand. With thumb, press a hole into centre of circle; pull dough apart to form a hole and smooth with fingers. Cover and let rise for 15 minutes.

In large stockpot bring water and sugar to boil. Turn down to medium heat. Gently place bagels in hot water (do only 2 or 3 at a time). Cook bagels for one minute. Turn and cook for 1 minute longer. Using slotted spoon, remove and drain briefly. Sprinkle non-stick or lightly greased baking pan with cornmeal. Place bagels on cornmeal and sprinkle with topping of your choice. Bake in 400°F (200°C) oven. When lightly brown, turn over. After about 20 to 25 minutes, when tops should be brown and sound hollow when tapped, remove from oven and place on metal rack to cool. If using glaze, combine egg white and water, brush over bagels.

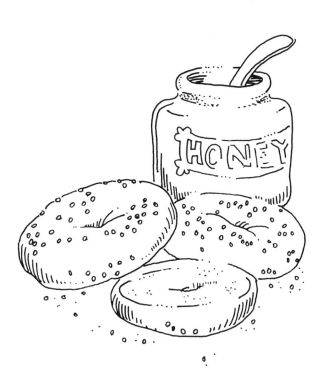

APRICOT BRAN BREAD
Maryanne Cattrysse, Simcoe, Ontario

Quick breads are extremely useful to have in the freezer and bring out for family or unexpected guests. Slices of this bran bread are wonderful served with a glass of milk for after school snacking or at tea time.

2 cups	bran cereal flakes	500 mL
½ cup	all-purpose flour	125 mL
½ cup	whole wheat flour	125 mL
½ cup	packed brown sugar	125 mL
2 tsp.	baking powder	10 mL
½ tsp.	salt	2 mL
½ tsp.	ground nutmeg	2 mL
¾ cup	chopped dried apricots	175 mL
1 tsp.	grated orange rind	5 mL
1	egg, lightly beaten	1
½ cup	skim milk	125 mL
½ cup	orange juice	125 mL
¼ cup	vegetable oil	50 mL

Loaf cakes slice more easily the next day. For best results, wrap loaf in foil; allow to stand overnight before slicing.

Preparation: 25 minutes
Cook: about 55 minutes
Makes 1 loaf or about 14 slices.

Calories per slice: 144
Grams of protein per slice: 2.7
Grams of fat per slice: 4.4
Grams of carbohydrate per slice: 24.8
Grams of fibre per serving: 1.9

Crush cereal to make ¾ cup (175 mL) crumbs. In large bowl, combine cereal, flours, sugar, baking powder, salt, nutmeg, apricots, and orange rind.

In second bowl, beat egg, milk, orange juice, and oil; stir into dry ingredients until well combined. Turn into non-stick or lightly greased 8 × 4-inch (1.5 L) loaf pan. Bake in 350°F (180°C) oven for about 55 minutes, or until tester inserted in centre comes out clean. Cool 10 minutes before removing from pan. Cool completely on wire rack.

STEAMED BROWN BREAD
Arlene Sturton, Ottawa, Ontario

This bread was made by our pioneer ancestors and is still a favourite today. This version is lower in sugar and higher in fibre than many brown bread recipes. It's great served with baked beans or a hearty soup for supper, or as a healthy after-school snack with cheese or peanut butter. You will need three 19-oz. (540 mL) fruit or vegetable cans or three coffee cans.

1 cup	all-purpose flour	250 mL
1 cup	whole wheat flour	250 mL
1 cup	cornmeal	250 mL
½ cup	granulated sugar	125 mL
1½ tsp.	salt	7 mL
1 tsp.	baking soda	5 mL
1½ cups	sour milk	375 mL
½ cup	molasses	125 mL
2 tbsp.	olive oil	25 mL

In large bowl, combine flours, cornmeal, sugar, salt, and baking soda.

In another bowl, combine sour milk, molasses, and olive oil. Add to dry ingredients, stirring just until moistened; do not overmix. Pour into 3 well-greased coffee cans; fill each about three-quarters full. Cover cans with foil; secure with elastic bands.

Into large Dutch oven or stockpot, bring about 4 cups (1 L) water to boil. Place coffee cans in water; cover and steam on low heat for 1½ to 2 hours. Remove cans from water and remove foil; allow to cool for 1 hour, or until tester inserted in centre comes out clean.

With a can opener, remove the bottom of the can and push the steamed bread through the open end. Leftovers may be frozen.

Preparation: 10 minutes
Cook: 1½ to 2 hours
Makes 3 loaves; about 10 slices per loaf.

Calories per slice: 82
Grams of protein per slice: 1.6
Grams of fat per slice: 1.2
Grams of carbohydrate per slice: 16.5
Grams of fibre per serving: 0.8

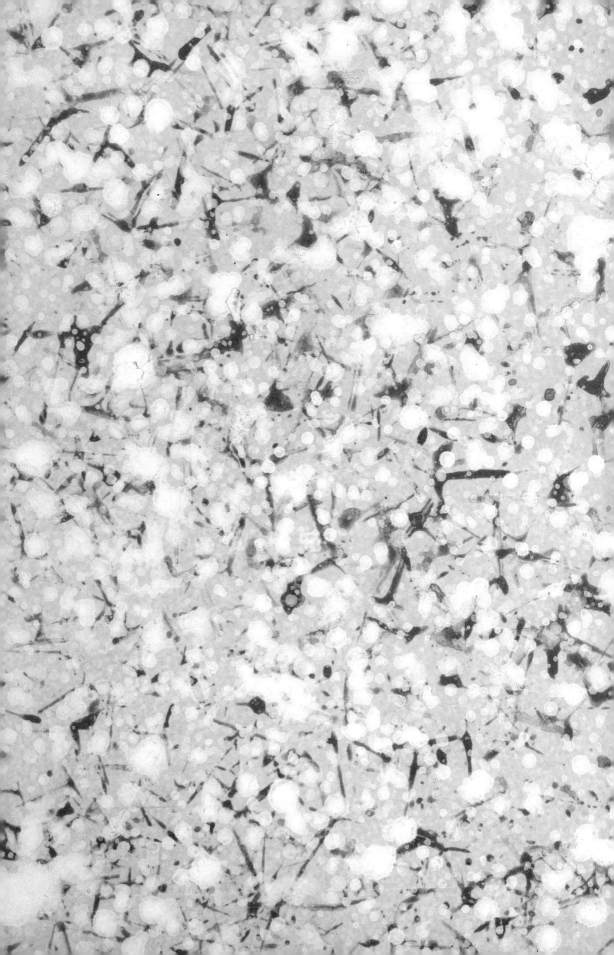

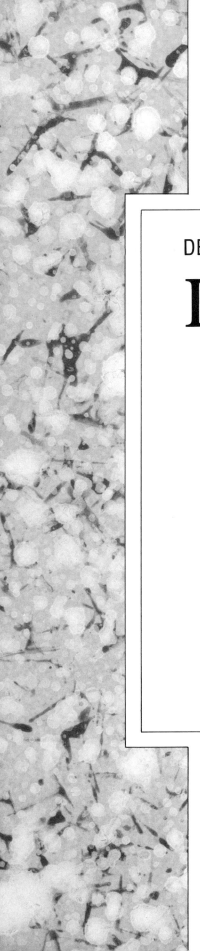

DELICIOUS   NEW   IDEAS   FOR

DESSERTS

Bet you never thought you'd hear a good word for desserts from dietitians. Well, like many popular generalizations, the notion that desserts are forbidden fruits is a gross exaggeration.

While it is true that the best sweet ending to a routine meal is fresh fruit, healthy eating does permit occasional indulgence—even downright decadence. In the case of desserts, the road to decadence is paved with fat and sugar—the more fat and sugar, the quicker the trip. But as is true elsewhere in life, moderation is all—and the recipes in this section illustrate how one can have the illusion of decadence without paying a devil's ransom.

"Sinfully delicious" is a term that can be applied even to food that is healthful and nutritious, as you will see in some of the winning recipes. Even more important is the fact that dessert can make a significant contribution to your daily nutrient requirements. So choose your food wisely, and enjoy the promise of a sweet treat to come!

SPIRITED FRUIT DESSERTS
Mary Sue Waisman, Calgary, Alberta

These desserts make perfect endings to heavier dinners.

PEARS IN PORT

1	orange	1
¼ cup	port wine	50 mL
4	firm pears, peeled, cored and halved	4

Makes 4 servings

Calories per serving: 134
Grams of protein per serving: 1.0
Grams of fat per serving: 0.7
Grams of carbohydrate per serving: 31.6
Grams of fibre per serving: 2.9

Peel orange. Cut peel into thin shreds. Squeeze juice from orange.

In large skillet, heat orange juice, port, and orange peel. Place pears in liquid; cook, uncovered, on low heat, basting at regular intervals, for about 20 minutes, or until pears are tender. Chill in liquid until serving time.

PEACHES AMARETTO
Combine 8 cups (2 L) peeled, sliced peaches with ½ cup (125 mL) amaretto liqueur. Cover and chill for 2 hours.

MARINATED MELON
Use 1 cup (250 mL) orange juice, ¼ cup (50 mL) lime juice, 2 tbsp. (25 mL) honey, and 1 tbsp. (15 mL) chopped fresh mint to marinate 2 cups (500 mL) each cantaloupe, watermelon, and honeydew balls.

NECTARINES IN COINTREAU
Poach sliced nectarines in light sugar syrup for about 5 minutes, or until they are tender. Allow to cool in syrup; pour some cointreau over fruit. Spoon syrup over fruit occasionally; serve chilled.

PINEAPPLE IN PORT
Peel, slice, and core a ripe pineapple. Place in large saucepan with grated peel of 1 orange and of ½ lemon, ½

If you've ever pondered over picking a pineapple, remember pineapples are harvested ripe. Unlike other fruit, they don't ripen after they're picked. Choose pineapples that look fresh, plump, and firm. Avoid ones with dry, brown leaves, bruises or an unpleasant odour. Store pineapple in a plastic bag in the refrigerator for three to five days.

cup (125 mL) granulated sugar, 1 cup (250 mL) pineapple juice, and ½ cup (125 mL) port. Simmer for 10 minutes; serve chilled.

SPICED BRANDIED CHERRIES
Fill sterilized pint jars with washed sour cherries. Add 1 cinnamon stick, 12 whole cloves, and ½ cup (125 mL) granulated sugar to each jar. Fill jar with brandy. Store for at least 3 months before using. Serve over sorbet, ice cream, or fresh fruit.

MELON WITH WINE
Cut a slice from stem end of large melon; scoop out seeds. Pour in ½ cup (125 mL) port, madeira, sherry, or a white dessert wine, like a sauterne. Replace slice. Refrigerate for several hours. Cut open and serve with wine juice from melon.

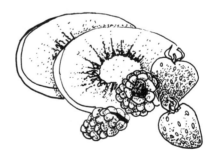

PEACHY UPSIDE-DOWN CAKE
Lois Eggert, Guelph, Ontario

This cake stores well in the refrigerator for up to 4 days. It is packed with fibre. Scatter a few blueberries between the sliced peaches as a variation.

1	can (14 oz./398 mL) sliced peaches, drained	1
	or	
2 cups	peeled and sliced fresh peaches	500 mL
⅓ cup	soft butter or margarine	75 mL
¾ cup	lightly packed brown sugar	175 mL
3	eggs	3
1½ cups	grated carrot	375 mL
¾ cup	whole wheat flour	175 mL
1¼ cups	high-fibre bran cereal	300 mL
1 tsp.	baking powder	5 mL
½ tsp.	baking soda	2 mL
½ tsp.	ground cinnamon	2 mL
¾ cup	raisins	175 mL

Drain peach slices thoroughly on absorbent paper. Arrange in bottom of 9-inch (23 cm) round cake pan lined with waxed paper. Set aside.

In large bowl, cream butter and sugar. Add eggs, one at a time, beating well after each addition. Stir in grated carrot.

In second bowl, combine flour, cereal, baking powder, baking soda, cinnamon, and raisins. Stir into carrot mixture. Spread evenly over peach slices. Bake in 350°F (180°C) oven for about 35 minutes, or until tester inserted in centre comes out clean. Let stand for 30 minutes before turning out onto serving plate. Serve warm or cold.

Preparation: 15 minutes
Cook: about 35 minutes
Makes 10 servings

Calories per serving: 251
Grams of protein per serving: 5.1
Grams of fat per serving: 8.0
Grams of carbohydrate per serving: 45.4
Grams of fibre per serving: 5.7

FRUITS FIT FOR A KING
Janice Ling, Scarborough, Ontario

The ingredients in this simple yet nutritious dessert can be a combination of favourite seasonal or exotic fruits, for example, kiwi fruit, mango, papaya, Japanese pear. However, several other fruits have been selected for their "light" taste and their availability.

TOPPING

½ cup	corn flakes or bran flakes, crushed	125 mL
¼ cup	unsalted shelled sunflower seeds	50 mL
1 tbsp.	wheat germ (optional)	15 mL

1 lb.	seedless green grapes	500 g
1 lb.	berries, such as strawberries	500 g
2	medium oranges, peeled and diced	2
1	medium apple, diced	1
1	medium pear, diced	1
1	medium peach or nectarine, diced	1
1 cup	Yorke Yoghurt (page 226) or low-fat plain yoghurt	250 mL

In large bowl, combine grapes, berries, oranges, apple, pear, and peach. Stir yoghurt into fruit and chill.

In separate bowl, combine corn flakes, sunflower seeds, and wheat germ. Spoon fruit and yoghurt mixture into small bowls; top with corn flake mixture.

MENU SUGGESTION
This is a light dessert that keeps calories and fat in check. Serve it after Iced Tomato Soup (page 64) and tarragon chicken salad on a Homemade Bagel (page 200) with romaine lettuce and sliced tomato for a meal with great taste, variety, and eye appeal. (Paula M. Fraser, R.Dt., St. John's, Newfoundland)

Preparation: 10 minutes
Chill: about 1 hour
Makes 6 servings

Calories per serving: 200
Grams of protein per serving: 4.8
Grams of fat per serving: 4.0
Grams of carbohydrate per serving: 40.8
Grams of fibre per serving: 5.2

For a wholesome dessert topping, try pureeing fruits such as strawberries, peaches, or raspberries in a blender or food processor. This dessert sauce is called a coulis. You don't need to add anything to the fruit. Spoon the coulis over other fruits, sherbets, ice cream, or cake. Use it as soon as possible after pureeing.

MENU SUGGESTION

The fruits in this fresh and pretty dessert offer a source of vitamins and fibre, but the biscuit baskets do add fat, so make your main course low in fat. Serve with a low-fat entrée such as Grape and Orange Sole Supreme (page 90) with a tossed green salad and low-fat dressing, brown rice, steamed green beans, and whole wheat roll. (Melanie Reeves, R.D., Calgary, Alberta)

BISCUIT BASKETS WITH BERRY COULIS
Goldie Moraff, Nepean, Ontario

Biscuit baskets, also known as French tuiles, are shaped like curved tiles (tuile being French for tile). They can be formed in two ways: over the bottom of a glass, or over a rolling pin. Keep some baskets in the freezer for last-minute serving of this "pretty as a picture" dessert.

BASKETS

⅔ cup	butter or margarine	150 mL
⅔ cup	granulated sugar	150 mL
1 cup	all-purpose flour	250 mL
2	egg whites	2
½ tsp.	almond extract	2 mL

COULIS

1	package (300 g) frozen unsweetened raspberries, thawed	1
1 tbsp.	Grand Marnier liqueur	15 mL
1 tsp.	granulated sugar	5 mL

FRUIT FILLING

4 cups	strawberries, sliced	1 L
2	kiwi fruit, peeled and sliced	2
½ cup	blueberries	125 mL
	Garnish: sweetened whipped cream, mint sprigs	

To make baskets: Cream butter and sugar. Beat in flour, egg whites, and almond extract. Set aside for 20 minutes.
Lightly grease eight 6-inch (15 cm) rounds of

The food stylist for this book, Jennifer McLagan, shared this tip on how to create a swirl effect in the coulis sauce. Drop about ½ tsp. (2 mL) whipping cream at intervals into the berry coulis sauce. Then with a wooden skewer or toothpick, draw a line of the cream through the purée. This technique helps you avoid using a large amount of whipping cream as a garnish.

Preparation: 30 minutes

Cook: about 7 minutes

Makes 8 servings

Calories per serving: 340

Grams of protein per serving: 3.6

Grams of fat per serving: 15.4

Grams of carbohydrate per serving: 48.6

Grams of fibre per serving: 3.1

parchment, foil, or brown paper. Spoon ¼ cup (50 mL) biscuit mixture into centre of each round. With a small spatula, spread dough thinly to cover the entire surface of each round.

Bake 2 rounds at a time on a baking sheet in 350°F (180°C) oven for about 7 minutes, or until slightly brown at the edges. Remove from oven; turn rounds over bottom of a glass and remove paper. Mould slightly to form a frilled edge. When cool, turn upright. Repeat for remaining biscuit rounds.

To make berry coulis: Strain raspberries through a sieve to remove seeds. Add liqueur and sugar to strained mixture.

To make fruit filling: Combine strawberries, kiwi fruit, and blueberries. Refrigerate until ready to serve.

To assemble: Place a small pool of berry coulis on one side of eight dessert plates. Place biscuit basket in middle of the plate and fill with prepared fruit. Garnish with whipped cream and mint sprigs.

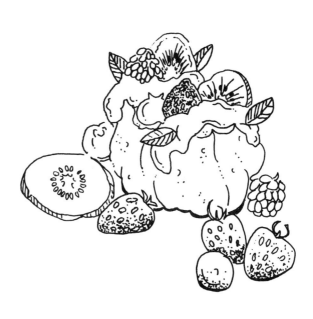

FRESH FRUIT WITH YOGHURT DRESSING

Elaine Watton, Corner Brook, Newfoundland

A refreshing and light salad dressing for a fruit salad plate or to drizzle over assorted fresh fruits for a dessert. Use any variety of your favourite fruits—oranges, apples, bananas, cantaloupe, pineapple, peaches, pears, or blueberries.

1 cup	low-fat plain yoghurt	250 mL
1 tbsp.	liquid honey	15 mL
1 tbsp.	freshly squeezed orange juice	15 mL
4 cups	cubed assorted fresh fruits	1 L
	Garnish: grated coconut	

Stir together yoghurt, honey, and orange juice. Place fruit in large bowl; pour yoghurt mixture over fruit. Refrigerate until serving time. Sprinkle with coconut.

Variation: To 1 cup (250 mL) Yorke Yoghurt (page 226), add 1 tbsp. (15 mL) freshly squeezed orange juice.

MENU SUGGESTION

This delightful combination of yoghurt and fresh fruit provides a clean fresh taste after a heavy meal. For a nutritious meal for family or friends that provides iron, niacin, vitamins A and C, and fibre while keeping down calories, serve spinach salad with herb vinaigrette, fish fillets with basil and lemon, parsley boiled new potatoes, and skillet zucchini with chopped tomatoes as a first course. (Paula M. Fraser, R.Dt., St. John's, Newfoundland)

Preparation: 10 minutes
Chill: 1 hour or longer
Makes 6 servings

Calories per serving of dressing: 36
Grams of protein per serving: 2.1
Grams of fat per serving: 0.6
Grams of carbohydrate per serving: 5.8
Grams of fibre per serving: 0

Calories per serving of dressing with fruit: 93
Grams of protein per serving: 2.8
Grams of fat per serving: 0.9
Grams of carbohydrate per serving: 20.3
Grams of fibre per serving: 1.8

ICY YOGHURT POPS

Barbara Hudec, Victoria, British Columbia

These refreshing popsicles are a nutritious alternative to sweeter frozen treats. Remove from the freezer to the refrigerator a few minutes before serving. Different flavours can be achieved by using a variety of puréed fruit or frozen fruit juice concentrates.

Popsicle trays can be bought in hardware stores or houseware departments.

Preparation: 10 minutes
Freeze: 2 to 3 hours or longer
Makes 6 to 7 servings

Calories per serving: 80
Grams of protein per serving: 3.3
Grams of fat per serving: 1.1
Grams of carbohydrate per serving: 14.7
Grams of fibre per serving: 0.2

1 cup	low-fat plain yoghurt	250 mL
¾ cup	frozen juice concentrate, thawed, or puréed fruit	175 mL
¾ cup	2 percent or skim milk	175 mL

Combine yoghurt, fruit juice concentrate, and milk. Pour into six or seven small paper cups. Freeze until partially frozen. Insert a wooden stick into centre of each; freeze until firm. To serve, peel off paper cup.

MENU SUGGESTION

A cool snack for kids and adults alike. Each pop provides calcium and has just one gram of fat. Serve for a schoolday lunch after Manitoba Vegetable Soup (page 62), peanut butter and banana sandwiches on whole wheat breads, and celery sticks. (Roxanne Eyer, Winnipeg, Manitoba)

PUMPKIN CUSTARD
Cynthia Chace, Dartmouth, Nova Scotia

Most baked custards have two or more eggs. This custard uses 2 percent evaporated milk and one egg for a slightly softer version of this comfort food.

Because of the risk of salmonella poisoning, raw eggs should be used with caution. Cracked eggs should be avoided. Recipes calling for raw eggs should be prepared as close to serving time as possible and kept well refrigerated.

1 cup	2 percent evaporated milk	250 mL
1 cup	canned or cooked mashed pumpkin	250 mL
2 tbsp.	granulated sugar	25 mL
1	egg	1
¼ tsp.	ground nutmeg	1 mL
¼ tsp.	ground ginger	1 mL

In blender or food processor, combine milk, pumpkin, sugar, egg, and spices. Process until well blended; pour into 4 large or 6 small custard cups. Bake in 325°F (160°C) oven for about 30 minutes, or until knife inserted in centre comes out clean. Serve warm or cold.

MENU SUGGESTION

This pumpkin custard is rich in calcium and vitamin A. It goes well after a main course of lean chicken breasts with brown rice and Winter Vegetable Salad (page 144) to complete a meal that provides fibre and controls fat. (Judith Creaser, P.Dt., Hantsport, Nova Scotia)

Preparation: 10 minutes
Cook: 30 to 35 minutes
Makes 4 to 6 servings

Calories per serving: 80
Grams of protein per serving: 4.4
Grams of fat per serving: 1.9
Grams of carbohydrate per serving: 11.8
Grams of fibre per serving: 0.4

Kiwi fruit was the fruit of the 1980s. It's now available year-round, thanks to New Zealand and California growers. Canada even has kiwi fruit growers on Vancouver Island! Wherever your kiwi fruit comes from, it'll ripen at home in 3 to 5 days at room temperature. Store ripe kiwi fruit in a plastic bag in the refrigerator for 2 to 3 weeks.

MENU SUGGESTION

The nuts are the main source of fat in this unique dessert, but they also contribute fibre. Keep the total amount of fat in balance with your other menu choices. Serve crudités with yoghurt dip, Vegetable Lover's Chili (page 103), and Steamed Brown Bread (page 203) for a first course. (Barbara Wunder, R.P.Dt., Toronto, Ontario)

Preparation: 15 minutes
Cook: 35 minutes
Makes 8 servings

Calories per serving: 229
Grams of protein per serving: 6.7
Grams of fat per serving: 10.3
Grams of carbohydrate per serving: 29.6
Grams of fibre per serving: 2.3

GERALDINE'S CAKE

Geraldine Mouyios, Regina, Saskatchewan

Guests will be sure to enjoy this nut torte with the unusual texture. If you serve it with fruit in season, you will not miss whipped cream. However, a small garnish can be piped on if desired.

4	eggs, separated	4
¾ cup	granulated sugar, divided	175 mL
¾ cup	rusk cracker crumbs (about 5 rusk crackers)	175 mL
¾ cup	ground almonds	175 mL
1 tsp.	vanilla extract	5 mL
½ tsp.	baking powder	2 mL
2 cups	seasonal fruit (kiwi fruit, blueberries, strawberries, raspberries, pineapple	500 mL

In large bowl, beat egg whites until soft peaks form. Gradually beat in ¼ cup (50 mL) sugar, beating well after each addition until sugar is dissolved and egg whites hold stiff, shiny peaks.

In second bowl, beat egg yolks with remaining sugar at medium speed until thick. Stir rusk crumbs, almonds, vanilla, and baking powder into egg-yolk mixture. Fold in beaten egg whites; pour into lightly greased 8-inch (20 cm) round pan. Bake in 350°F (180°C) oven for about 35 minutes, or until cake springs back when touched. Let stand 10 minutes; remove cake from pan; allow to cool on wire rack. Serve topped with fresh fruit.

FLUFFY PUMPKIN CHEESECAKE
Judy Koster, Bridgewater, Nova Scotia

You can make this creamy, mellow cheesecake year-round using canned pumpkin with this spicy gingersnap crumb crust.

CRUST

1 ½ cups	gingersnap crumbs	375 mL
⅓ cup	melted butter or margarine	75 mL
3 tbsp.	firmly packed brown sugar	45 mL

FILLING

1 cup	unsweetened apple juice	250 mL
⅔ cup	granulated sugar	150 mL
½ tsp.	salt	2 mL
1	envelope unflavoured gelatine	1
3	eggs, separated	3
½ tsp.	vanilla extract	2 mL
1	package (250 g) cream cheese	1
1 tbsp.	lemon juice	15 mL
¾ cup	whipping cream	175 mL
¼ tsp.	ground cloves	1 mL
¼ tsp.	ground cinnamon	1 mL
¼ tsp.	ground ginger	1 mL
1 cup	canned or cooked mashed pumpkin	250 mL
	Garnish: semi-sweet chocolate curls (optional)	

MENU SUGGESTION

Although this is a high-fat dessert (60 percent of the calories come from fat), it is so delicious that we had to include this recipe in our book. But balance the meal by serving it after a low-fat main course of baked boneless chicken breast without the skin, brown rice, and steamed vegetables. A good idea would be to serve it on a day when your physical activity is high. (Jeanne McCutcheon, R.D.N., Richmond, British Columbia)

To make crust: Combine gingersnap crumbs, butter, and brown sugar. Press on bottom and sides of 9-inch (23 cm) springform pan. Refrigerate while preparing filling.

Photos: Biscuit Baskets with Berry Coulis, page 210 (facing page); Icy Yoghurt Pops, page 213 (overleaf)

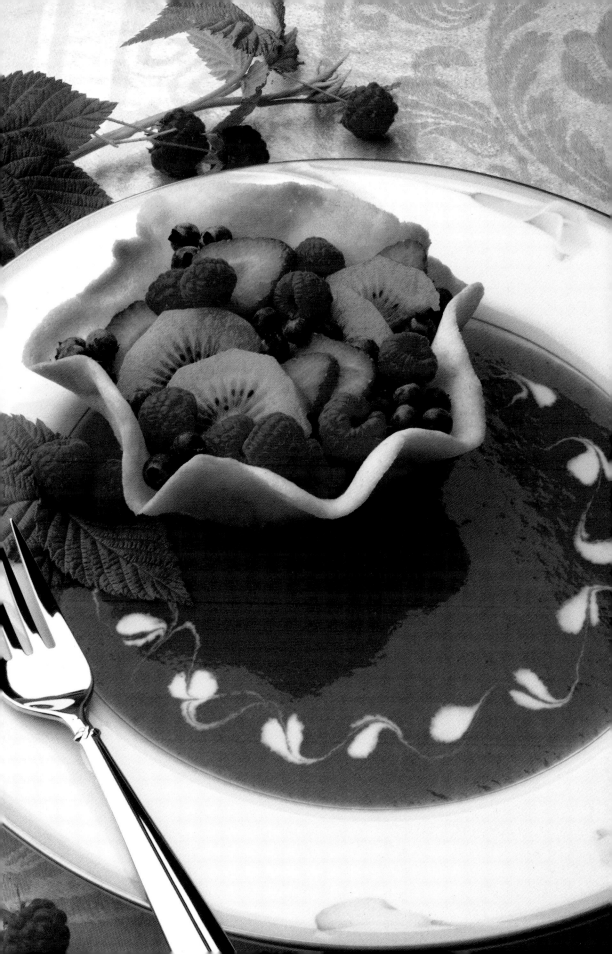

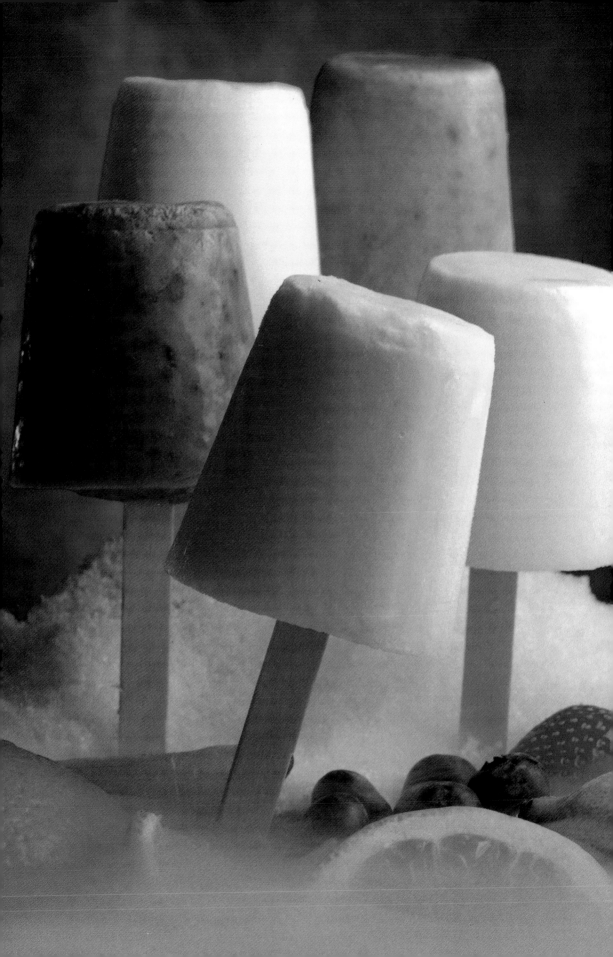

To make filling: In small saucepan, combine apple juice, sugar, and salt. Sprinkle gelatine over apple juice. Cook over low heat, stirring constantly, for 3 minutes, or until gelatine is completely dissolved.

Beat egg yolks slightly. Gradually stir in some hot liquid; return to saucepan. Cook on medium heat, stirring constantly, for about 5 minutes, or until thickened. Stir in vanilla.

With an electric mixer, combine cream cheese, and lemon juice. Add gelatine mixture; beat on high speed until smooth. Chill until mixture is consistency of unbeaten egg whites, about 30 minutes.

Beat egg whites until stiff. In a separate bowl, combine cream and spices; beat until stiff. Fold whipped cream, pumpkin, and egg whites into gelatine mixture. Pour into springform pan; chill for about 3 hours, or until firm. Garnish with chocolate curls before serving.

Preparation: 30 minutes
Chill: 3 hours or longer
Makes 12 servings

Calories per serving: 296
Grams of protein per serving: 4.7
Grams of fat per serving: 19.5
Grams of carbohydrate per serving: 27.0
Grams of fibre per serving: 0.4

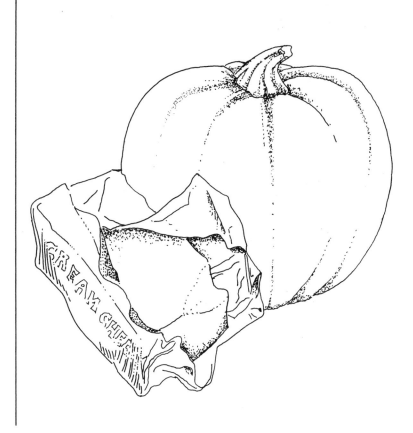

STRAWBERRY YOGHURT PIE
Kellogg Canada Inc.

A fluffy filling with a crunchy crust makes this pie a light refreshing ending to a special meal. This recipe is best when served the same day it is made.

CRUST

3 tbsp.	butter or margarine	45 mL
3 tbsp.	corn syrup	45 mL
3 tbsp.	firmly packed brown sugar	45 mL
2½ cups	bran flakes cereal	625 mL

FILLING

1	package (85 g) strawberry gelatine	1
1 cup	boiling water	250 mL
1	package (300 g) frozen unsweetened whole strawberries, slightly thawed	1
1 cup	low-fat plain yoghurt	250 mL

To make crust: In saucepan on medium-high heat, melt butter, corn syrup, and brown sugar; bring mixture to full boil, stirring continuously. Remove from heat; stir in cereal, mixing until cereal is completely coated. Press firmly around sides and bottom of lightly greased 9-inch (23 cm) pie plate. Place in freezer while preparing filling.

To make filling: Dissolve gelatine in boiling water. Cut strawberries into small pieces; stir into jelly mixture. Chill until mixture reaches the consistency of egg whites. Whisk in yoghurt. Chill briefly until mixture is thick but not set. Pour into chilled pie crust. Refrigerate about 2 hours before serving.

Variation: This recipe can also be made with unsweetened raspberries, which would increase the fibre content to 4.4 g per serving. Substitute fresh berries when available.

MENU SUGGESTION

Another dessert that can serve as a light finish to a meal. The fat is kept to a minimum and the cereal-based crust contributes fibre. Serve after a meal of Barbecued Stuffed Salmon (page 88), Tarragon Vinaigrette Potato Salad (page 142), green beans almandine, and Blond Sangria (page 238). (Mary Ellen MacDonald, R.P.Dt., Guelph, Ontario)

Preparation: 30 minutes
Chill: 2 hours or longer
Makes 8 servings

Calories per serving: 199
Grams of protein per serving: 4.3
Grams of fat per serving: 4.9
Grams of carbohydrate per serving: 37.3
Grams of fibre per serving: 2.6

CINNAMON BAKED PEARS IN YOGHURT SAUCE

Christine Cauch, Downsview, Ontario

Poaching fruit in cinnamon syrup results in flavour saturation. Pears are not the only fresh fruit that can be prepared in this manner. Consider peaches, nectarines, apples, fresh pineapple, or oranges.

4	medium pears	4
½ cup	blueberries	125 mL
½ cup	water	125 mL
2 tbsp.	lightly packed brown sugar	25 mL
1 tbsp.	lemon juice	15 mL
¼ tsp.	ground cinnamon	1 mL

YOGHURT SAUCE

½ cup	low-fat plain yoghurt	125 mL
1 tbsp.	lightly packed brown sugar	15 mL
½ tsp.	ground cinnamon	2 mL
½ tsp.	vanilla extract	2 mL

For added fibre, leave the skin on pears, apples, peaches, and nectarines.

Preparation: 15 minutes
Cook: about 45 minutes
Makes 4 servings

Calories per serving: 167
Grams of protein per serving: 2.3
Grams of fat per serving: 1.2
Grams of carbohydrate per serving: 40.1
Grams of fibre per serving: 3.3

Peel pears and cut in half lengthwise; scoop out core. Place cut side down in shallow baking dish. Sprinkle blueberries around pears.

Combine water, brown sugar, lemon juice, and cinnamon; pour over pears. Bake, covered, in 350°F (180°C) oven for about 45 minutes, or until pears are tender. Baste pears occasionally with pan juices.

To prepare sauce: In small bowl, combine yoghurt, brown sugar, cinnamon, and vanilla.

Serve pears with pan juices; spoon a dollop of yoghurt sauce over cooked pear halves.

MERINGUE FRUIT TORTE
Joyce Gillelan, Weston, Ontario

This meringue, as light as a cloud, may be filled with a lemon sauce and seasonal fruit — blueberries, raspberries, strawberries, peaches — or tropical fruits. Meringues can be prepared ahead and stored for up to 1 week, providing they are kept in a tightly sealed container. Make either 1 large or 6 individual meringues.

MERINGUE

2	egg whites, at room temperature	2
½ tsp.	white vinegar	2 mL
Pinch	salt	Pinch
½ cup	granulated sugar	125 mL

LEMON SAUCE

⅔ cup	granulated sugar	150 mL
2 tsp.	cornstarch	10 mL
1 tsp.	grated lemon peel	5 mL
⅓ cup	water	75 mL
⅓ cup	fresh lemon juice	75 mL
1	egg, beaten	1
2 cups	cut-up fresh fruit	500 mL
	Garnish: Mint leaves	

To make meringue: In bowl, combine egg whites, vinegar, and salt. Beat until soft peaks form. Add sugar, 1 tbsp. (15 mL) at a time; beat until stiff peaks form.

Line a baking sheet with parchment or brown paper (aluminum foil may also be used). Draw a circle with an 8-inch (20 cm) diameter. Spoon egg-white mixture on paper pattern; with a spoon shape mixture into a circle with sides about 2 inches (5 cm) higher than centre. Or prepare individual meringues 2 inches (5 cm) in diameter.

Bake single meringue in 250°F (120°C) oven for about 1½ hours, or until slightly coloured. Turn off oven and leave meringue to cool for 2 hours or overnight before removing from oven. Carefully remove from paper. (Bake individual meringue for 50 to 60 minutes).

To make lemon sauce: In small saucepan, combine sugar, cornstarch, and lemon peel. Stir in water and lemon juice; cook over medium heat, stirring constantly until slightly thickened. Carefully stir one-quarter of hot mixture into beaten egg to prevent egg from coagulating; return to hot mixture, stirring constantly. Cook and stir for 4 minutes, or until thickened. Cover and refrigerate.

Just before serving, combine cut-up fruit with lemon sauce. Spoon into meringue shell and serve, garnished with mint leaves.

Serve this zesty lemon sauce over plain cake, Hot Water Gingerbread (page 233), milk pudding, fresh fruit, or fruit sherbet like Strawberry Sorbet (page 223). Angel cake, hollowed out, is an alternative to meringue shell.

Preparation: 1 hour
Cook: 1½ hours
Makes 6 servings

Calories per serving: 192
Grams of protein per serving: 2.5
Grams of fat per serving: 1.1
Grams of carbohydrate per serving: 45.1
Grams of fibre per serving: 1.0

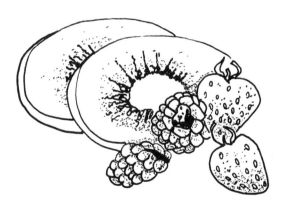

WINTER FRUIT CRISP

Laurie A. Wadsworth, Swift Current, Saskatchewan

Several fruits make a crisp more colourful and add extra flavour. Depending on the natural sweetness of each fruit, more or less sugar may be required. Large-flake rolled oats give that old-fashioned crunchy topping we all remember.

3	large apples, peeled and sliced	3
2	large pears, peeled and sliced	2
½ cup	cranberries, fresh or frozen	125 mL
2 tbsp.	granulated sugar	25 mL
1 cup	large-flake rolled oats	250 mL
¼ cup	brown sugar	50 mL
¼ cup	natural wheat bran	50 mL
½ tsp.	ground cinnamon	2 mL
⅓ cup	butter or margarine	75 mL

Place apples, pears, and cranberries in shallow baking pan. Sprinkle with sugar.

In medium bowl, combine oats, brown sugar, bran, and cinnamon. With pastry blender or two knives, cut in butter until crumbly. Sprinkle over fruit mixture.

Bake in 400°F (200°C) oven for about 40 minutes, or until mixture is bubbling and fruit is barely tender.

MENU SUGGESTION

This dessert, with its fibrous crunchy topping, is an excellent finish to a meal of braised Cornish hens, wild rice with mushrooms, mixed vegetables, and tossed salad with low-cal dressing. (Madge Ma, P.Dt., Saskatoon, Saskatchewan)

Preparation: 15 minutes
Cook: 40 minutes
Makes 6 servings

Calories per serving: 293
Grams of protein per serving: 3.1
Grams of fat per serving: 11.4
Grams of carbohydrate per serving: 49.3
Grams of fibre per serving: 5.7

STRAWBERRY SORBET
Vicki McKay, Woodstock, Ontario

The popularity of low-fat sorbets is on the increase. Make this with raspberries, peaches, blueberries, kiwi fruit, cantaloupe or other fruits.

1½ cups	fresh or frozen unsweetened strawberries	375 mL
2 cups	unsweetened apple juice	500 mL
¼ cup	granulated sugar	50 mL
¼ tsp.	ground cinnamon	1 mL
2 tbsp.	cold water	25 mL
4 tsp.	cornstarch	20 mL

Wash and hull fresh strawberries or thaw frozen strawberries. In blender or food processor, blend strawberries and apple juice until almost smooth.

In medium saucepan over medium heat, cook strawberry mixture, sugar, and cinnamon, stirring frequently, for about 5 minutes, or until sugar is dissolved. Combine water and cornstarch; stir into hot mixture. Cook for about 3 minutes, or until thickened and clear. Chill for 1 hour. Pour into 8-inch (2 L) square pan; cover and freeze for about 3 hours, or until firm.

Break frozen mixture into chunks; beat with electric mixer at medium speed until fluffy. Transfer to an airtight container and freeze until firm. Remove from freezer to refrigerator about 15 minutes before serving.

MENU SUGGESTION

This sorbet, which contributes vitamin C, is the perfect low-fat ending to any meal. For a simple yet elegant dinner, serve it as dessert after chilled cucumber and yoghurt soup, lemon herbed barbecued chicken breasts, wild rice, and Deluxe Peas (page 125). (Yolanda Jakus, R.P.Dt., London, Ontario)

Preparation: 10 minutes
Chill: 1 hour
Freeze: about 3 hours
Makes 6 servings

Calories per serving: 85
Grams of protein per serving: 0.3
Grams of fat per serving: 0.2
Grams of carbohydrate per serving: 21.3
Grams of fibre per serving: 1.0

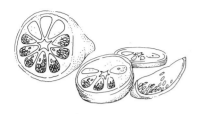

LEMON SHERBET
Joan Gallant, Newcastle, New Brunswick

This is similar to a frozen soufflé, but is lighter and lower in calories. Everyone on the taste panel gave this a very high rating.

½ cup	granulated sugar	125 mL
⅓ cup	lemon juice	75 mL
2 tsp.	grated lemon rind	10 mL
2	eggs, separated	2
⅔ cup	skim-milk powder	150 mL
⅔ cup	cold water	150 mL

Whisk together sugar, lemon juice, rind, and egg yolks; set aside.

With an electric mixer, beat egg whites, skim-milk powder, and water on high speed for 3 to 5 minutes, or until stiff peaks form. Fold in lemon mixture. Pour into 8 small custard cups; cover and freeze for about 3 hours, or until firm. Remove from freezer to refrigerator about 15 minutes before serving.

MENU SUGGESTION

This light, low-calorie dessert complements any meal. For a varied menu that keeps calories in check, serve Vegetable Bouillon Break (page 240), Barbecued Stuffed Salmon (page 88), hearty bread, broccoli spears, and carrot coins, with Lemon Sherbet for dessert. (Joy Johns, P.Dt., Saint John, New Brunswick)

Preparation: 10 minutes
Freeze: about 3 hours
Makes 8 servings

Calories per serving: 88
Grams of protein per serving: 3.5
Grams of fat per serving: 1.4
Grams of carbohydrate per serving: 15.9
Grams of fibre per serving: 0

PINEAPPLE FRUIT PLATE WITH DIP
Mrs. F.R. Smith, Winnipeg, Manitoba

Light cream cheese is used to make this luscious dip for a fresh fruit plate, or topping for cut-up fresh fruit. Serve it as an appetizer on a hot summer day, or as a light finish to a heavier meal any time.

MENU SUGGESTION
You can take advantage of the fresh fruits in season to make this recipe different every time you serve it. Local blueberries, strawberries, or saskatoons will add fibre to your diet. Remember that sauces and dips increase total fat, so don't overdo it. This dessert will complement a meal of romaine lettuce with Raspberry Basil Vinaigrette (page 153), bread sticks, Manitoba smoked goldeye, wild rice, and asparagus with lemon sauce. (Wanda Smith-Windsor, R.D., Selkirk, Manitoba)

Preparation: 15 minutes
Cook: 10 minutes
Chill: 2 hours
Makes about 1 cup (250 mL) dip
Serving size: 1 tbsp./15 mL

Calories per serving: 39
Grams of protein per serving: 1.2
Grams of fat per serving: 1.6
Grams of carbohydrate per serving: 4.9
Grams of fibre per serving: 0

Makes 6 servings of fruit and dip
Serving size: ¾ cup/175 mL

Calories per serving: 156
Grams of protein per serving: 4.0
Grams of fat per serving: 4.8
Grams of carbohydrate per serving: 25.9
Grams of fibre per serving: 1.4

4½ cups	Fresh pineapple cubes; watermelon, cantaloupe or honeydew balls; red or green grapes; blueberries, raspberries, or strawberries	1.1 L

DIP

½ cup	unsweetened pineapple juice	125 mL
¼ cup	granulated sugar	50 mL
1 tbsp.	cornstarch	15 mL
1 tbsp.	lemon juice	15 mL
1	egg, beaten	1
1	package (125 g) light cream cheese	1
	Garnish: fresh mint leaves	

Refrigerate fruit.

In small saucepan over medium heat, cook pineapple juice, sugar, cornstarch, and lemon juice, stirring constantly, for about 5 minutes, or until clear and thickened. Slowly stir some hot mixture into beaten egg. Return to saucepan and cook over low heat until mixture thickens slightly. Cool for 5 minutes. Whisk in cream cheese until smooth. Refrigerate for at least 2 hours, or until very cold, before serving with fresh fruits. Garnish with mint.

YORKE YOGHURT
Kathryn Yorke, Winnipeg, Manitoba

For yoghurt-lovers without a yoghurt-maker, this recipe will come in very handy. A low-fat, inexpensive version, it uses skim-milk powder and the heat from an oven light to set the yoghurt overnight. The yoghurt will be slightly less firm than commercial yoghurt. When a plain yoghurt is required for other recipes in the book, omit honey.

2½ cups	skim-milk powder	625 mL
5½ cups	cold water	1.4 L
3 tbsp.	low-fat plain yoghurt	45 mL
3 tbsp.	liquid honey (optional)	45 mL

In large Pyrex or ceramic bowl, whisk together skim-milk powder and water. Microwave on High (100 percent) about 5 minutes, or until hot, or scald in large saucepan on medium heat. Cool to room temperature.

Whisk in yoghurt. Place in cool oven overnight with oven light left on. In the morning, whisk in honey and refrigerate.

Orange Yoghurt Dessert

Mary Malerby, Vernon, British Columbia combines 4 peeled and diced oranges with 2 cups (500 mL) Yorke Yoghurt and ¾ tsp. (4 mL) coconut extract and chills. This dessert serves 4.
Calories per serving: 128
Grams of protein per serving: 6.2
Grams of fat per serving: 0.3
Grams of carbohydrate per serving: 26.9
Grams of fibre per serving: 3.1

Preparation: 10 minutes
Makes about 6 cups (1.5 L)

Calories per cup: 133
Grams of protein per cup: 10.0
Grams of fat per cup: 0.3
Grams of carbohydrate per cup: 23.1
Grams of fibre per cup: 0

What grows upside down, comes neatly packaged, and is available year round? The banana! This tropical fruit ripens best after harvesting. If your bananas are ripe, you can keep them from further ripening by putting them in the refrigerator for a few days. The peel will turn black but inside the fruit will be fine.

CRANBERRY SURPRISE
Laura M. Hawthorn, Bracebridge, Ontario

This is one of two cranberry recipes Laura Hawthorn sent to us. She lives in an area where cranberries are grown locally and uses them in this recipe and in her Cranberry Oat Muffins (page 193).

2 cups	graham cracker crumbs	500 mL
½ cup	butter or margarine, melted	125 mL
2 cups	2 percent milk	500 mL
1	package (92 g) cooked-style vanilla pudding*	1
2 cups	fresh or frozen cranberries, chopped	500 mL
1	large banana, mashed	1
½ cup	granulated sugar	125 mL
¼ cup	chopped nuts (walnuts, pecans, or almonds)	50 mL

Combine graham cracker crumbs and butter. Press two-thirds of crumb mixture onto bottom of 8 × 12-inch (3 L) baking pan. Bake in 325°F (160°C) oven for 10 minutes. Remove pan from oven and let cool on rack.

Cook milk and vanilla pudding according to package directions; allow to cool for about 15 minutes.

Combine cranberries, banana, and sugar; set aside.

Spread cooked pudding over crumb base. Top with cranberry mixture. Sprinkle with remaining crumbs and chopped nuts. Refrigerate for 4 to 5 hours.

MENU SUGGESTION

With its high fat content, this dessert should be reserved for days when your overall fat intake is low. It would go well after a meal of Confetti Pork (page 95), rice, and broccoli spears with lemon. (Ellen van der Meer, R.P.Dt., Owen Sound, Ontario)

---

* Instead of milk and pudding, you could make a homemade cornstarch milk pudding like the filling for Strawberry Coconut Supreme (page 228).

Preparation: 20 minutes
Chill: 4 to 5 hours
Makes 9 to 12 servings

Calories per serving: 240
Grams of protein per serving: 3.5
Grams of fat per serving: 11.4
Grams of carbohydrate per serving: 34.0
Grams of fibre per serving: 1.5

What's the best way to ripen fruit after you buy it? Place the fruit in a paper bag, loosely close it, and put the bag on top of your refrigerator, or in any warm spot. Don't use an air-tight plastic bag for ripening, as it will cause the fruit to sweat, which promotes spoilage.

STRAWBERRY COCONUT SUPREME
Sandra L. Schultz, Luseland, Saskatchewan

This dessert, made with fresh fruit and coconut, has a tropical flair. It is elegant but easy to make ahead of time.

CRUST

1 cup	graham cracker crumbs	250 mL
3 tbsp.	melted butter or margarine	45 mL

CUSTARD FILLING

2 cups	2 percent milk, divided	500 mL
⅓ cup	granulated sugar	75 mL
1	egg, slightly beaten	1
⅓ cup	finely shredded coconut	75 mL
3 tbsp.	cornstarch	45 mL
1 tsp.	coconut extract or vanilla extract	5 mL

TOPPING

1½ cups	sliced strawberries	375 mL

MENU SUGGESTION
This delightful summertime dessert is a delicious way to finish a meal, but remember to plan for it. It contains a significant amount of fat and calories, so cut down on your other fat sources during the day. Serve it after lamb shish kebabs, barbecued potatoes, green beans with Herb Tomato Salad Dressing (page 154), and warm pita bread. (Helene Machnee, P.Dt., Saskatoon, Saskatchewan)

Preparation: 25 minutes
Chill: 1½ hours
Makes 6 servings

Calories per serving: 258
Grams of protein per serving: 5.4
Grams of fat per serving: 11.5
Grams of carbohydrate per serving: 35.5
Grams of fibre per serving: 2.8

To make crust: Combine graham cracker crumbs and butter. Press onto bottom of 8-inch (2 L) square pan. Bake in 325°F (160°C) oven for 10 minutes. Remove pan from oven and let cool on rack.

To make filling: In medium saucepan over medium heat, bring to a boil 1½ cups (375 mL) milk, sugar, egg, and coconut; stir occasionally. Combine cornstarch with remaining milk; stir into hot milk; cook, stirring constantly, until mixture is thickened. Remove from heat; stir in coconut extract. Cool for 10 to 15 minutes and pour over crumb mixture. Refrigerate for at least 1½ hours.

At serving time, arrange sliced strawberries over pudding.

CARROT PIE

Laure Riendeau, Longueuil, Quebec

Pumpkin pie lovers will also enjoy this French-Canadian specialty. Carrots provide a pleasing texture and appearance. The filling is thin but sets nicely during baking.

PASTRY FOR SINGLE CRUST 9-INCH (23 CM) PIE

2 cups	thinly sliced carrots	500 mL
2	eggs, lightly beaten	2
1 cup	2 percent milk	250 mL
½ cup	granulated sugar	125 mL
1 tsp.	ground cinnamon	5 mL
1 tsp.	ground nutmeg	5 mL
½ tsp.	ground ginger	2 mL
¼ tsp.	salt	1 mL

Line pie plate with pastry; chill while preparing filling.

Cook carrots until tender; drain well and purée. Beat eggs, carrot, milk, sugar, and spices. Pour into prepared pie shell.

Bake in 425°F (220°C) oven for 10 minutes. Reduce heat to 350°F (180°C) and bake for about 35 minutes longer, or until tester inserted in centre comes out clean. Serve warm or at room temperature.

MENU SUGGESTION

This dessert has almost 13 grams of fat per slice, so keep the fat in the rest of the meal to a minimum. It is certainly a new way to eat your vegetables. Serve it after a main course of roast pork with apple and raisin stuffing, baked potatoes topped with yoghurt and herbs, Braised Cabbage (page 124), and whole wheat rolls. (Jane McDonald, R.Dt., St. John's, Newfoundland)

Preparation: 15 minutes
Cook: 45 minutes
Makes 6 servings

Calories per serving: 278
Grams of protein per serving: 5.6
Grams of fat per serving: 12.9
Grams of carbohydrate per serving: 35.7
Grams of fibre per serving: 1.7

MARBLE CHIFFON CAKE WITH CHOCOLATE FUDGE ICING
Lenore Ramos, Winnipeg, Manitoba

This feather-light dessert is wonderful on its own or frosted with Chocolate Fudge Icing. By omitting the cocoa mixture in the cake recipe, you will have a Golden Chiffon Cake, which can be served with sliced fresh fruit, or iced with a Caramel Frosting (recipe below).

CHOCOLATE FUDGE ICING (OPTIONAL)

¼ cup	butter or margarine	50 mL
2	squares unsweetened chocolate	2
1	can (300 mL) sweetened condensed milk	1

MENU SUGGESTION

This cake has 7 grams of fat per slice even without icing, so go easy on the fat for the rest of the meal. Serve it after consommé, Turkiaki Fiesta (page 83), brown rice, pineapple spears, and skim milk. (Ellen Vogel, R.D., Winnipeg, Manitoba)

¼ cup	unsweetened cocoa	50 mL
¼ cup	hot water	50 mL
1¾ cups	all-purpose flour	425 mL
1½ cups	granulated sugar	375 mL
1 tbsp.	baking powder	15 mL
1 tsp.	salt	5 mL
½ cup	safflower oil or sunflower oil	125 mL
5	eggs, separated	5
¾ cup	water	175 mL
2 tsp.	vanilla extract	10 mL
½ tsp.	cream of tartar	2 mL

Combine cocoa and hot water; set aside.

In large bowl, combine flour, sugar, baking powder, and salt. In separate bowl, mix together oil, egg yolks, water, and vanilla. Stir into dry ingredients; beat for 2 minutes, or until smooth.

In small bowl, beat egg whites until foamy; add cream of tartar and beat until stiff peaks form. Fold beaten whites into flour mixture. Remove half of batter into separate bowl; fold in cocoa mixture. Pour both batters into a non-stick or lightly greased 10-inch (3 L) tube pan. Gently run spatula through batter to give a marbled effect. Bake in 325°F (160°C) oven for 55 minutes. Increase temperature to 350°F (180°C); bake 10 minutes longer, or until cake springs back when lightly touched.

Invert cake in pan on a rack until cool. Remove to serving plate. Frost with Chocolate Fudge Icing or simply dust with sifted icing sugar. Cake freezes well.

To make Chocolate Fudge Icing: In saucepan over low heat, melt butter and chocolate with condensed milk; cook, stirring constantly, for about 5 minutes, or until thickened (it will thicken quickly). Cool slightly before spreading on cake.

CARAMEL FROSTING
(Submitted by Alice Mullin, Sault Ste. Marie, Ontario)
In small saucepan over low heat, melt ¼ cup (50 mL) butter or margarine. Stir in ½ cup (125 mL) packed brown sugar and 2 tbsp. (25 mL) 2 percent milk. Bring to boil, stirring constantly. Remove from heat. Stir in 1 cup (250 mL) sifted icing sugar and 1 tsp. (5 mL) vanilla extract until spreading consistency. Frost Golden Chiffon Cake (Marble Chiffon Cake can be made without cocoa mixture) and sprinkle with ¼ cup (50 mL) chopped nuts.

Preparation: 15 minutes
Cook: about 1 hour
Makes 16 to 20 servings

Calories per serving without icing: 167
Grams of protein per serving: 2.9
Grams of fat per serving: 7.1
Grams of carbohydrate per serving: 23.8
Grams of fibre per serving: 0.3

Calories per serving with icing: 262
Grams of protein per serving: 4.7
Grams of fat per serving: 12.1
Grams of carbohydrate per serving: 35.7
Grams of fibre per serving: 0.3

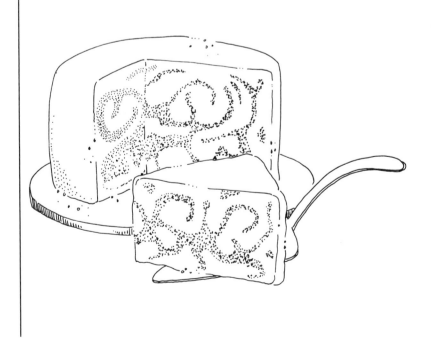

LEMON PUDDING

Valerie Caldicott, Powell River, British Columbia

*This is a less sweet version of an old-fashioned family favourite.
What's old is new again!*

1	medium lemon	1
⅓ cup	granulated sugar	75 mL
2 tbsp.	all-purpose flour	25 mL
Dash	salt	Dash
2	eggs, separated	2
1 cup	2 percent milk	225 mL

With a lemon zester or grater, remove rind from lemon.
Squeeze juice; set juice and rind aside.

In mixing bowl, combine sugar, flour, and salt. Stir in
lemon juice, rind, beaten egg yolks, and milk. Beat egg
whites until stiff but not dry; fold into lemon mixture.

Pour into lightly greased 4-cup (1 L) baking dish. Place
in larger pan, pour in hot water to about 1-inch (2.5 cm)
depth. Bake in 350°F (180°C) oven for about 30 minutes,
or until topping is set and golden brown. Serve warm.

Preparation: 15 minutes
Cook: about 30 minutes
Makes 4 servings

Calories per serving: 150
Grams of protein per serving:
5.5
Grams of fat per serving: 4.0
Grams of carbohydrate per
serving: 23.6
Grams of fibre per serving: 0.1

HOT WATER GINGERBREAD
Mary Sue Waisman, Calgary, Alberta

This old-fashioned family dessert is a real comfort food. Serve warm with Lemon Sauce (page 220), a light custard sauce, or freshly prepared unsweetened apple sauce.

1½ cups	all-purpose flour	375 mL
1 tsp.	baking soda	5 mL
1 tsp.	ground ginger	5 mL
½ tsp.	ground cinnamon	2 mL
¼ tsp.	salt	1 mL
1	egg	1
½ cup	firmly packed brown sugar	125 mL
½ cup	molasses	125 mL
½ cup	boiling water	125 mL
⅓ cup	melted butter or margarine	75 mL

In large bowl, combine flour, baking soda, and seasonings.

In second bowl, beat egg, brown sugar, molasses, and boiling water. Stir molasses mixture and melted butter into flour mixture until well blended. Pour into non-stick or lightly greased 8-inch (2 L) square baking pan. Bake in 350°F (180°C) oven for about 35 minutes.

Preparation: 15 minutes
Cook: 35 minutes
Makes 9 servings

Calories per serving: 224
Grams of protein per serving: 2.9
Grams of fat per serving: 7.3
Grams of carbohydrate per serving: 37.1
Grams of fibre per serving: 0.6

LAZY DAISY CAKE
Camille Morris, Edmonton, Alberta

Many of you may remember your mother or grandmother making this light, sponge-style cake. Prepare and store in the freezer for last-minute desserts or for peach, raspberry, or strawberry shortcake.

2	eggs	2
1 cup	granulated sugar	250 mL
1 tsp.	vanilla extract	5 mL
1 cup	all-purpose flour	250 mL
1 tsp.	baking powder	5 mL
Pinch	salt	Pinch
½ cup	2 percent milk	125 mL
2 tsp.	butter or margarine	10 mL

In medium bowl, beat together eggs, sugar, and vanilla until light and fluffy.

Combine flour, baking powder, and salt; set aside.

Scald milk; stir in butter until melted. Add to egg mixture alternately with flour mixture, beginning and ending with flour.

Pour batter into 8-inch (2 L) non-stick or lightly greased round baking pan. Bake in 350°F (180°C) oven for about 35 minutes, or until tester inserted in centre comes out clean. Allow to cool on wire rack for 10 minutes before removing from pan.

Preparation: 10 minutes
Cook: 35 minutes
Makes 9 servings

Calories per serving: 163
Grams of protein per serving: 3.3
Grams of fat per serving: 2.2
Grams of carbohydrate per serving: 32.8
Grams of fibre per serving: 0.4

BUTTERMILK OAT-BRANANA CAKE
Helen Sutton, Sudbury, Ontario

The glaze poured over this cake makes it extra moist and delicious. The panel awarded the honourable mention in the dessert category of the Healthy Eating Recipe Contest to this fabulous cake.

GLAZE

½ cup	granulated sugar	125 mL
½ cup	buttermilk	125 mL
¼ cup	butter or margarine	50 mL
½ tsp.	baking soda	2 mL

1 cup	buttermilk	250 mL
⅔ cup	rolled oats	150 mL
⅓ cup	oat bran or wheat bran	75 mL
¼ cup	butter or margarine	50 mL
1 cup	granulated sugar	250 mL
1	egg	1
1 tsp.	vanilla extract	5 mL
2	ripe bananas, mashed	2
1½ cups	all-purpose flour	375 mL
1 tsp.	baking soda	5 mL
1 tsp.	baking powder	5 mL

MENU SUGGESTION

This tasty cake is a hearty accompaniment that adds additional fibre to a soup meal. Serve it following a meal of Fish and Vegetable Medley (page 68), cucumber vinaigrette, and wholewheat bread. (Jeanine Chaisson, R.Dt., St. John's, Newfoundland)

In small bowl, pour buttermilk over rolled oats and oat bran. Let stand for 10 minutes.

In medium bowl, cream butter and sugar. Beat in egg and vanilla. Combine bananas and buttermilk-oat mixture with creamed ingredients. Sift together flour, baking soda, and baking powder. Stir dry ingredients into banana mixture; blend well.

Pour batter into lightly greased and floured 8-inch (2 L) square cake pan. Bake in 350°F (180°C) oven for 45 minutes, or until tester inserted in centre comes out clean. Let stand 5 minutes.

Meanwhile prepare glaze. In small saucepan over medium heat, combine sugar, buttermilk, butter, and baking soda. Bring just to boil. (Watch closely, mixture will foam.) Makes approximately 2 cups (500 mL) glaze.

Poke holes with tester (a metal skewer or a wooden toothpick) all over cake surface; pour glaze over cake while still warm. Cool cake before cutting.

Preparation: 20 minutes
Cook: 45 minutes
Makes 8 generous servings or 12 smaller servings

Calories per serving: 277
Grams of protein per serving: 4.5
Grams of fat per serving: 8.8
Grams of carbohydrate per serving: 46.3
Grams of fibre per serving: 1.5

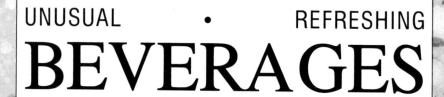

UNUSUAL • REFRESHING

BEVERAGES

Try some of these interesting combinations to add variety to your meals and entertaining. These drinks can be bright new accompaniments to your own favourite recipes or to the recipes in this book.

E ven the beverages you choose can make a nutritional contribution to your day. You are probably already drinking milk, juices, and water. Here are some new ways of combining these beverages with fruits, vegetables, and spices. Try to keep alcohol and caffeine to a minimum.

The fresh cranberry season is very short. You can extend the life of your cranberry by freezing this tangy, North American berry. To freeze, pop the fresh cranberries, exactly as they come from the store, right into your freezer. When you want to use them, simply rinse the frozen berries. No thawing is necessary. Use them in any recipe that calls for fresh cranberries.

HOT MULLED CRANBERRY JUICE
Kelly and Barbara Waddingham, Brockville, Ontario

This is the perfect drink to warm you up after any cold-weather activity.

4 cups	cranberry juice	1 L
4	dried apricot halves	4
2 tbsp.	chopped fresh or frozen cranberries	25 mL
2 tbsp.	raisins	25 mL
4	whole cloves	4
1	cinnamon stick	1
Pinch	ground nutmeg	Pinch
	Garnish: Cinnamon sticks	

In large non-aluminum saucepan, combine cranberry juice, apricots, cranberries, raisins, cloves, cinnamon stick, and nutmeg. Heat, covered, on medium high for about 10 minutes, or until heated through; remove cloves and cinnamon stick. Serve warm with a cinnamon stick if desired.

Variation: Amber rum may be added.

Preparation: 10 minutes
Cook: 10 minutes
Makes 4 to 5 servings

When entertaining, be sure to have non-alcoholic beverages as a choice for your guests. You can perk up your non-alcoholic drinks by preparing ice cubes made of pieces of fresh fruit and juice. As the ice cubes melt, they add flavour to the drink. Frozen fruit molds also add a special touch when added to punches.

BLOND SANGRIA

Kelly and Barbara Waddingham, Brockville, Ontario

Sangria is typically made using red wine. This lighter, more refreshing version is a perfect party punch for summer and is prepared with chilled white grape juice or white wine. Sangrias are always more flavourful when fruit and juices are allowed to marinate for several hours or overnight.

1	bottle (750 mL) dry white wine, chilled or	1
3 cups	white grape juice, chilled	750 mL
1	bottle (750 mL) apple juice, chilled	1
¼ cup	lime juice	50 mL
1 cup	sliced green seedless grapes	250 mL
1	orange, sliced and quartered	1
1	lime, cut into thin wedges	1
1	bottle (750 mL) club soda, chilled	1
	Ice Ring	

To eliminate dilution of punch, use apple juice in ice ring.

Combine wine or grape juice, apple and lime juices, grapes, orange slices and lime wedges; marinate in refrigerator until serving time.

Just before serving, place wine mixture in punch bowl; add club soda and ice ring.

To make ice ring: To prevent cloudiness in ice ring, boil and chill the water. Fresh fruit or flowers may be placed in bottom of mould and frozen in a shallow layer of boiled water; then add more water and freeze for several hours or until required.

Preparation: 15 minutes
Marinate: several hours or overnight
Makes about 14 cups (3.5 L) or 25 servings

TROPICAL FRUIT SLUSH

Lena (Barrett) Putnam, Winsloe, Prince Edward Island

Serve this on those dog days of summer when the temperature is high.

1½ cups	peeled and chopped peaches or nectarines	375 mL
½ cups	peeled and chopped mango or papaya, or sliced strawberries	375 mL
½ cup	water	125 mL
2 tsp.	lime juice	10 mL
½ tsp.	coconut extract	2 mL
1 cup	pineapple juice	250 mL
	Garnish: lime wedge	

Preparation: 15 minutes
Freeze: 2 to 3 hours
Makes 4 cups (1 L) or 4 to 6 servings

In blender, combine peaches, mango, water, lime juice, coconut extract, and juice. Process until smooth. Pour into flat pan; cover and freeze for 2 to 3 hours, or until slushy. Spoon into 4 glasses. Garnish with lime wedge.

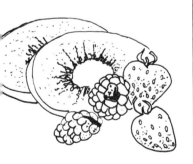

BERRY SHAKE

Shelley Moffat, Calgary, Alberta

2 cups	skim milk	500 mL
1 cup	fresh or frozen raspberries or strawberries	250 mL
1 tbsp.	liquid honey	15 mL
½ cup	low-fat plain yoghurt	125 mL
	Garnish: whole raspberries or strawberries	

Preparation: 10 minutes
Makes about 2½ cups (625 mL) or 2 servings

In blender, process milk and berries until very smooth; strain if using raspberries. Return to blender; add honey and yoghurt; process for about 15 seconds or until fluffy. Pour into chilled glasses.

VEGETABLE BOUILLON BREAK
Eleanor Jackson, Toronto, Ontario

Enjoy as a change from mid-morning coffee or with a sandwich at lunch.

1 cup	water	250 mL
1 cup	vegetable juice cocktail	250 mL
1 tbsp.	lemon juice	15 mL
½ tsp.	beef bouillon powder	2 mL
¼ tsp.	dried thyme	1 mL
Dash	hot pepper sauce	Dash
	Garnish: 2 lemon slices	

Preparation: 5 minutes
Cook: 5 minutes
Makes 2 cups (500 mL) or 2 servings.

In small saucepan, heat water, vegetable cocktail, lemon juice, beef bouillon, and seasonings until hot. Pour into mugs; serve with lemon slices.

HOT CURRIED TOMATO JUICE
Bernie Warden, Calgary, Alberta

Bernie Warden, a friend of one of the authors, shared this recipe for a pleasant warm accompaniment to a sandwich at lunch.

2	green onions	2
2 cups	tomato juice	500 mL
2 tsp.	curry powder	10 mL
	Freshly ground pepper	
¼ cup	low-fat plain yoghurt	50 mL

Preparation: 15 minutes
Cook: 5 minutes
Makes 2 cups (500 mL) or 2 to 3 servings.

Cut white part from green onions; reserve green part. Finely chop white part; combine with tomato juice and seasonings in small saucepan. Cook until heated through.

In blender, combine hot tomato mixture and yoghurt; quickly process until smooth. Pour into mugs; serve hot garnished with green onion stalks.

SPARKLING PEACH BELLINI
Ron Morris, Montreal, Quebec

This punch is festive enough for a wedding party punch or open house.

2½ cups	water	625 mL
1	can (6 oz./170 mL) frozen concentrated orange juice, thawed	1
1	bottle (750 mL) champagne or white wine chilled	1
1	bottle (750 mL) sparkling mineral water chilled	1
1	can (12 oz./355 mL) peach nectar, chilled	1
	Garnish: orange or peach slices, optional	

In large punch bowl, combine water, orange juice, champagne, mineral water, and peach nectar; stir well. Garnish with orange slices to float. Serve immediately.

For single servings, Ron Morris splashes a small quantity of white wine over the peach nectar in a glass to thin the nectar. He then tops the glass with champagne. The orange juice and mineral water are omitted in this version.

Preparation: 10 minutes
Makes 12 cups (3 L) or about 16 servings.

ACKNOWLEDGMENTS

The Canadian Dietetic Association would like to thank many people whose hard work made this book possible.

First of all, a hearty thanks to Helen Bishop MacDonald, who wrote the healthy eating chapters, and to her husband, Sandy MacDonald, for his support. Also many thanks to Margaret Howard for screening, testing, and refining the many consumer recipes, and to her husband John Howard for his support.

Thanks are also extended to those who worked on the preparation and presentation of the recipes: Janet Baillie, Kay Dallimore, Lois Eggert, Joyce Gillelan, Shirley Ann Holmes, Shelley Moffat, Marilyn Smith, and Brenda Steinmetz.

John Howard and Paul Howard did the computer data entry and Sharyn Joliat, R.P.Dt., of Info Access, Toronto, did the nutrient analyses.

We'd also like to thank all those who reviewed the book or participated in the taste panels: Anne Birks, Dorothy Boothe, Evelyn Carter, Christine Cauch, Michele Cauch, Pauline Cauch, Lisa Famularo, Handzia Feloniuk, Marion Glumac, Mathew Hurd, Aiden Kelly, Dave Kirkland, Christine Kunicki, Jacynte LeRoux, Janine MacLachlan, Karen Massari, Sharon Parker, Halia Radiuk, Diane Robb, Bob Romanyk, Linda Ruscio, Cynthia Rutherford, Rene Schoepflin, Susan Sedlbauer, Diane Shearman, Andrea Silva, and Colin Wackett.

Thanks also to the many dietitians who contributed to the development of the book with critical review or input: Denise Beatty, R.P.Dt., Nutrition Expressions, King City, Ontario; Dr. Elizabeth Bright-See, R.P.Dt., University of Western Ontario, London, Ontario; Susan Close, R.P.Dt., Waterloo Regional Health Unit, Kitchener, Ontario; Doris Gillis, P.Dt., Antigonish, Nova Scotia; Helen Haresign, R.P.Dt., Director, Public Relations, The Canadian Dietetic Association; Tammy Hirose, R.D., Calgary General Hospital, Calgary, Alberta; Shelagh Kerr, R.P.Dt., Grocery Products Manufacturers of Canada, Toronto, Ontario; Mary Ellen MacDonald, R.P.Dt., Guelph, Ontario; Marsha Sharp, R.P.Dt., Executive Director, The Canadian Dietetic Association; Susan Sutherland, R.P.Dt., Fresh for Flavour Foundation, Ottawa, Ontario; Cheryll Tucker, R.P.Dt., Notre Dame of St. Agatha, St. Agatha, Ontario; Ellen Vogel, R.D., Department of Health, City of Winnipeg, Winnipeg, Manitoba; Mary Sue Waisman, R.D., Chair, National Nutrition Campaign Steering Committee, The Canadian Dietetic Association, Calgary, Alberta; Dr. Donna Woolcott, R.P.Dt., University of Guelph, Guelph, Ontario.

Thanks also to the many dietitians across Canada who developed menus for the recipes.

Thanks to the staff of the following sponsors for their input: Grissol, Kellogg Canada Inc., Kraft General Foods, the Dairy Bureau of Canada, and the Ontario Milk Marketing Board. And finally, thanks to the staff of GCI Communications, Toronto, Ontario, for their coordination.

Photo Credits

Photography: Fred Bird, photographer; Jennifer McLagen, food stylist; Debby Boyden, props; and David Field, photo assistant, all of Toronto, Ontario.

Photography Props

Thanks to Bronson's China and Gifts, Toronto, Ontario, for supplying props for the following photographs: Turkiaki Fiesta (white plate); Biscuit Baskets with Berry Coulis (plate and fork); Babsi's Broccoli Soup (bowl and spoon); West Coast Chicken Salad (plate); Mixed Greens with Fresh Strawberries (glass bowl); Deluxe Peas (bowl and spoon); Spaghetti Squash with Mushrooms (plate and utensils); Cottage Cheese-Filled Crêpes (glasses and china); Fish Fillets with Basil Walnut Sauce (platter); Ginger-Vegetable Beef Medley (plate).

Thanks also to the Pottery Shop, Toronto, Ontario, for supplying props for the following photographs: Oriental Crab Spread and Lemon Pesto Spread (ceramics); Falafel and Tabbouleh (black plate); Cheesy Broccoli and Potato Casserole (casserole dish).

INDEX